Hearing Impaired Infants:
Support in the First Eighteen Months

Hearing Impaired Infants: Support in the First Eighteen Months

Edited by
Jacqueline Stokes

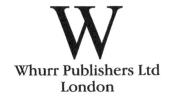

Whurr Publishers Ltd
London

© 1999 Whurr Publishers
First published 1999 by
Whurr Publishers Ltd
19b Compton Terrace, London N1 2UN, England

Reprinted 1999, 2001 and 2002

Exclusively distributed in North America by
Paul H. Brookes Publishing Company, P.O. Box 10624,
Baltimore, Maryland 21285-0624

British Library Cataloguing in Publication Data
A catalogue record for this book is available from the
British Library.

ISBN: 1 86156 106 7

Printed and bound by CPI Antony Rowe, Eastbourne
Reprinted 2006

Contents

Foreword

Children who are seriously hearing impaired cannot acquire language without special help. Without effective language and good communication skills, they cannot be expected to learn in school. Without effective schooling throughout childhood, limited personal, social and employment opportunities are available in life.

Few parents are aware of the effects of serious deafness because it is an uncommon disability, only about one child in a thousand being affected. Such parents find that many of the professionals involved often disagree about how best to provide optimal help for these children. Many current conflicts among professionals, perhaps more particularly those using sign rather than spoken language, arise because the ongoing advances in research and technology challenge traditional and well-established educational methods. Such advances have led to radically improved opportunities for the acquisition of natural spoken language. Such recent developments, discussed in this text in a straightforward, easy-to-read manner, have helped to open the way for family members to become more actively and effectively involved in hearing impaired children's overall development. Parents, as this book shows, are now more widely encouraged than ever before to assume a full and active partnership with various professionals as members of the child's management team. Indeed, parents are increasingly recognized as the most essential agents in the development of their children's communication skills.

This is a timely book, for when change is evident, there is usually some resistance to it that calls for careful examination. The authors, several highly successful and well-respected professionals, show that some such resistance is justified – for rational decisions relating to a child's future cannot be made if the potentials of change are not fully understood. They know at first hand how current developments can affect children who are hearing impaired. They provide well-informed, well-balanced information that highlights the importance of individual differences between children, differences that preclude any one form of education as suitable for meeting the needs of them all. At the same time, the authors skilfully guide readers through the maze of conflicts that are commonly met by parents and professionals who are newcomers to the field. This is a book that will help many parents and professionals to avoid the development of communicative and educational deficits in children that are unfortunately (and often unnecessarily) associated with hearing loss in the early years of life.

Daniel Ling PhD
Professor Emeritus
University of Western Ontario, Canada

Preface

A tremendous amount of work is involved in the diagnosis and subsequent management of a young child with a permanent sensorineural hearing loss. This process involves both professionals from health and education services *and* parents.

The central importance of parents is noted in a recent National Deaf Children's Society Quality Standards document:

> Parents should be regarded as full members of the team supporting the hearing-impaired child, alongside professionals. Optimal habilitation occurs only in situations where parents are valued as equal members of a well coordinated and accessible team. (Quality Standards in Paediatric Audiology, Vol. 2, 1996).

But we still do not have a clear idea of what it means to have parents as equal members of the team. Many pay lip service to this ideal, but little has been done to translate this theory into practice. The purpose of this book is to share information about this work among all those involved.

Experience shows that when it comes to treating children, professionals and parents do not share the same language. In particular, they each perceive issues differently. This book is written by professionals who have long experience of working in active co-operation with parents and who allow the voice of the parents to come through clearly. The purpose of this book is twofold. First, we aim to convey, in a clear and readable manner, what we as professionals do, the language we use, those elements which aid decision-making and some of the ramifications of hearing impairment. The benefit to parents from using this book is that they will be in a better position to formulate the child's needs and ensure these are met. Second, most of us, as professionals, have not had the harrowing experience of discovering that our child has a hearing impairment, and we can learn from parents about the full impact of living 24 hours a day with a child who does not hear well. This, in turn, should lead us to become more sensitive and understanding professionals.

Teams work best when each member supports the work of all the other team members. It is essential therefore that everyone involved in the team understands what the other members are trying to achieve. This book is also intended for parents and all professionals wanting to support the hearing impaired child and his family.

In the first chapter of the book, Roger Green goes straight to the crux of the matter and explains what we mean by 'Your child has a hearing loss'. To do this, he describes how ears work, what can go wrong and how we measure hearing in babies and young children. One of the first questions parents ask when faced with the diagnosis of hearing loss in their child is, 'What is the cause?' In Chapter 2, Valerie Newton and I give an overview of the major causes of hearing loss and outline some of the investigations that help to determine the cause. It is crucially important to the family to understand the factors that caused the hearing loss in their child. This chapter emphasizes the benefit of making timely referrals for appropriate investigations, co-ordinating results and counselling parents throughout the process.

Once a permanent hearing loss has been identified and medical or surgical treatment has been ruled out, the next issue to be raised is that of hearing aids. In Chapter 3, Roger Green describes the art of fitting hearing aids to small children at a time when their parents are still dealing with the impact of the diagnosis. He covers a range of technical detail that is important in understanding the types of aids available, how they work and how they are selected. His skill is in never losing sight of the fact that the patient is a child first and foremost, and the challenge to the paediatric audiologist is to make the technology work for each child and his family.

In Chapter 4, Roger Wills continues with this theme as he looks at those children who are found to have mild and moderate hearing losses. These children are frequently born with a hearing problem that is not confirmed until they are 2 or 3 years old. The lateness of the diagnosis may lead to a variety of problems, such as understanding how the hearing loss was overlooked as well as the guilt that many parents feel in accepting hearing aids. There is a tendency to misunderstand and underestimate this degree of hearing loss. A child with a mild or moderate hearing loss is not 'severely' or 'profoundly' impaired, yet his parents may grieve for the loss and worry about his future in the same way as parents of children with more severe losses.

Wendy Lynas tackles the central problem that faces parents: which communication method is best for my child? Everyone seems to have a view on this question, and opinions can quickly become entrenched and extreme. In her chapter on Communication Options, Wendy presents the arguments and the evidence for three different communication methods. This chapter gives a balanced view so that parents can begin to find a communication option with which they feel comfortable. It also challenges all professionals to think critically about the communication issue and to reconsider their assumptions about the 'best' method.

The cochlear implant is a remarkable development in hearing aid technology. It is a device that bypasses the damaged part of the ear and directly stimulates the hearing nerve. It provides parents with another option for their profoundly deaf child when conventional hearing aids are found wanting. Elizabeth Tyszkiewicz and Jo Edwards have worked in a children's cochlear implant centre for many years and are experienced at talking and listening to parents as they weigh the pros and cons of cochlear implants. In Chapter 6, they describe the process of cochlear implantation from referral to an implant centre through to the integration of the device into the child's life.

In Chapter 7, Sue Lewis looks at another worrying dilemma for parents: 'Where will my child go to school?' She describes the variety of school placements that are available nationally and discusses the advantages and disadvantages of each. From her experience as an educational consultant and OFSTED trained schools inspector, she is able to give parents insight into the kinds of question they should ask when considering school placement options. This chapter brings us right up to date with the current legislative position and provides parents and professionals with a considerable amount of practical, useful information on the statementing process and parental involvement.

In the concluding chapter, all the various issues are brought together using one particular child, Chloe, as a case study. The chapter illustrates how the diagnosis, the investigations of the cause, the hearing aid fitting, the development of communication and finding a school all interlink to provide effective and appropriate family support.

The book is meant to provide a tool for teaching, learning and working with hearing impaired children. It is not intended to provide a 'cookbook' approach to the early management of hearing impairment, nor is it meant to be prescriptive about one method in favour of another. Instead, the aim is to give parents enough information to make effective choices, to build their confidence so that they can secure the most appropriate support and encouragement for their infant.

In order to reach these diverse audiences, we have tried to produce a book that is readable, jargon-free and straightforward, and which includes a wealth of practical information. The reference and further reading lists provide signposts towards finding out more information for readers who wish to pursue one particular subject in more detail.

For the sake of simplicity, when singular pronouns were necessary in our writing, we have used the masculine form. This decision should not be viewed as discriminatory but as an effort to avoid the repetitive introduction of awkward constructs such as he/she.

This book is the collective effort of individuals who are trying, from a variety of angles, to meet some of the ideals expressed by organizations such as the National Deaf Children's Society. Drawing on the collective skills and experience of the distinguished team of authors assembled in this book, we hope that the content will facilitate closer working relationships between everyone involved in the complex, unpredictable and emotional business of trying to meet the needs of children who are hearing impaired.

Jacqueline Stokes
Audiology Department
Royal Berkshire Hospital
Reading

Acknowledgements

I would like to begin by acknowledging Daniel Ling, who first got me hooked on working with families and hearing impaired children. Others who have given sound advice and useful criticism during the preparation of the manuscript include Sue Miller, Morag Clark, Judy Hortt, Susan Cassingham and Roger Wills. My thanks also go to Steve Woolgar and Alexandra, Madeleine and Francesca, who have provided endless support and encouragement. Finally, on behalf of all the authors, I wish to express our sincere thanks to all the children and families who have contributed to our understanding of families and hearing impairment.

Jacqueline Stokes
Wolvercote
September 1998

Contributors

Jo Edwards Audiologist, Manchester Paediatric Cochlear Implant Programme, Central Manchester Healthcare NHS Trust

Roger Green Clinical Director of Audiology, King Edward VII Hospital, Windsor

Sue Lewis Educational Consultant for the Ewing Foundation, Centre for Human Communication and Deafness, University of Manchester

Wendy Lynas Senior Lecturer, Education of the Deaf, Centre for Human Communication and Deafness, University of Manchester

Valerie Newton Professor of Audiological Medicine, Centre for Human Communication and Deafness, University of Manchester

Jacqueline Stokes Early Language Adviser in Audiology, Royal Berkshire Hospital, Reading

Elizabeth Tyszkiewicz Co-ordinator, Manchester Paediatric Cochlear Implant Programme, Central Manchester Healthcare NHS Trust, University of Manchester

Roger Wills Principal Audiological Scientist, Royal Berkshire Hospital, Reading

Chapter 1
Audiological identification and assessment

ROGER GREEN

Photographs by Joanne Lazenby

What do you mean, my child can't hear?

It can be devastating for parents to be told for the first time, 'Your child is deaf': What does it mean? Why has it happened? What did we do wrong? Will he ever speak? Will he have to go to a special school? How do we talk to him? What do we do? Why us? Why our child? Parents are suddenly catapulted into a world about which they had, up until that point, no knowledge and probably not a lot of interest.

In the midst of the emotional turmoil, they somehow have to cope with a whole new world of ideas and terms. Furthermore, the knowledge that they need has to be conveyed to them by clinicians who have been 'doing it for years' and who may have some difficulty putting themselves in the parents' shoes. Yet the parents are the key figures in the process of helping their child. Knowledge is part of their armoury, and it is the clinicians' responsibility to help them gain that knowledge. It is a process that requires patience, sensitivity and flexibility, going at the right pace, frequently revisiting issues the clinician may have assumed were already covered, treading a convoluted path to understanding. What the clinician takes for granted may leave the parent very confused. I remember being brought up sharply by a parent of a 1-year-old child who was several months into wearing hearing aids when he simply asked one day, 'Why fit hearing aids to a child who can't hear?'

So, what do we mean, 'Your child can't hear'? This simple question underlies the whole complexity of human hearing. We now need to explore the process of hearing, in terms of how ears work, what can go wrong and how we can measure hearing.

Everyone is different

The senses of hearing and seeing are our two most developed senses. Much of our communication is through hearing. We can hear friends and family

1

speaking to us, and our own replies. We can hear music. We can hear when there is someone knocking at the door or calling on the telephone. We can hear the warning sounds of an approaching car or a fire alarm. We can even tell where things are coming from (a skill we possess from having two ears).

So will a deaf child have none of this? There is an all-or-nothing misunderstanding about the term 'deafness' – the misunderstanding that a child is either normal, in which case he can hear everything (the sound of his mother's voice, the dog barking downstairs, a car turning into the driveway) or a child is deaf, in which case he can hear nothing.

In fact, total deafness is very rare. Most children who have hearing loss still have some hearing. Indeed, a hearing loss can be anything from mild to profound. Hearing loss can also be temporary or permanent. Some children may hear some sounds quite normally and other sounds only when they are loud enough. For example, a child might hear all sounds except for high-pitched ones. He may hear low-frequency sounds (the rumble of a plane overhead, the bang of a door-knocker, the vowel sounds in speech) quite well, even normally. However, he may not hear high-frequency sounds (the squeak of a toy, the ringing of a tele-phone, consonant sounds in speech) at all. To him, the world can still sound a noisy place, but sounds will be blurred or muffled. People will sound as if they are talking through cotton wool.

Other children may have more severe losses. For some children, all they can hear is an 'island' of low-pitched sounds, and they can only hear these when they are made very loud. They will hear virtually nothing useful (except perhaps a very loud 'NO!' when on the point of emptying their dinner onto the carpet).

It should be clear then that deafness varies, and deaf children are not all the same. Exactly what they hear depends on what has gone wrong.

How ears work – anatomy and physiology

So what can go wrong? Parents need to understand deafness in terms of what has happened in the ear (and sometimes the rest of the hearing system). There are many books that deal with the ear and how it works, and the reader is referred to these if he or she wishes to know more. This section will attempt only an outline summary of the ear and hearing system, but this will hopefully be enough to give an initial understanding of the hearing system and how it can fail.

We can divide the ear into five sections:

Outer ear • Middle ear • Inner ear • Nerve of hearing • Brain.

The outer ear

The outer ear comprises the pinna and ear canal. The pinna has the job of catching sound and steering it down the ear canal towards the

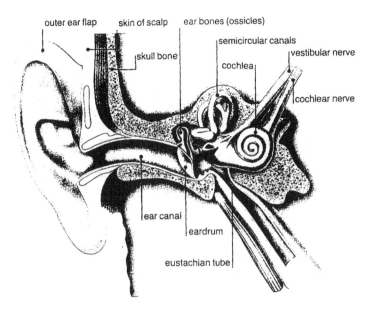

outer ear flap   skin of scalp   ear bones (ossicles)

semicircular canals

skull bone   vestibular nerve

cochlea

cochlear nerve

ear canal

eardrum

eustachian tube

Figure 1.1 Diagram of the ear.

eardrum. The ear canal is surprisingly long, so the drum is well protected deep within the skull. It is almost level with the back of the eye, about 2.5 cm into the head. It is in the ear canal that earwax forms. Wax is a useful substance, catching dirt and debris that gets into the ear. The wax is gradually pushed out by tiny hairs in the ear canal, until it reaches the canal entrance and flakes away.

The middle ear

The middle ear is made up of the eardrum, ossicles and middle ear space. The eardrum closes the ear canal off from the middle ear – one reason why you do not fill up with water when you go swimming! The middle ear is a small, air-filled cavity behind the eardrum. Connected to the eardrum are three tiny bones (the smallest in the body), which act as a bridge, carrying the sound across the middle ear cavity to the inner ear.

Another important feature is a small tube that connects the middle ear to the back of the throat. This is called the Eustachian tube. The Eustachian tube allows air into the middle ear, equalizing the pressure with the air outside. This is important because the ear is designed to work best when the pressures on both sides of the eardrum are equal. If the tube fails to work properly, for example when you have a cold, the ears may start to feel blocked. It is very common for children to have Eustachian tube problems, and this can lead to the condition known as glue ear, which is described below.

The inner ear

The last small bone in the chain carries the sound across to the inner ear, or cochlea. Inside this 'snail shell' structure is a complex network of many thousands of tiny sound-sensitive cells, immersed in fluid. The cells are called hair cells because of small hairs protruding from the top of each of them. The hair cells pick up the vibrations from the ear bones and convert them into nerve signals (rather like a solar panel changing light into electricity). The process is a complex one, but the important thing to understand is that the hair cells have the job of translating the mechanical vibrations entering the cochlea into nerve signals that the brain can understand.

The nerve of hearing

The nerve of hearing connects the cochlea to the brain. The nerve signals, which are really just tiny electrical impulses, are carried from the back of the cochlea by a bundle of tiny fibres (as in an electrical cable).

The brain

The brain is an interesting place. There is no single part of the brain where all incoming 'sounds' are finally analysed. As the nerve of hearing passes into the lower brain, or brainstem, it divides into many branches, which spread across the entire brain. Many of these branches finish up on the other side of the brain. In other words, many of the signals from the left ear go to the right side of the brain, and those from the right ear to the left side of the brain. From there they spread to many other areas of the brain.

What can go wrong – pathology

Conductive deafness and sensorineural deafness

Problems with the outer and middle ears cause what is called 'conductive' deafness. This is because the problem lies in the mechanism that conducts sound to the cochlea. It is often possible to correct conductive deafness with medicine or surgery.

Problems with the inner ear or nerve of hearing cause what is called 'sensorineural deafness' (sometimes called nerve deafness, although this term is confusing when the damage is to the hair cells in the cochlea rather than to the nerve of hearing). It is not usually possible to correct sensorineural deafness with medicine or surgery.

The outer ear

Wax is much misunderstood. Excessive wax in the ear canal causes at worst a very slight hearing loss, yet it is often the first thing people blame. It is virtually never the main cause of significant childhood deafness.

The principal cause of hearing loss from the outer ear is a problem called canal atresia. In this condition, the child is born without an ear canal. Instead of the canal there is bone or cartilage preventing the sound from getting through to the cochlea. If both ears show atresia, a special 'bone conduction' hearing aid can help. Some children with atresia may eventually be able to have an operation that clears the blocked ear canals. In such cases, the hearing aids are fitted as a temporary measure.

The middle ear

By far the most common cause of hearing loss in children comes from fluid building up in the middle ear space behind the eardrum. This condition takes several forms and goes by many names, the most common of which is 'glue ear'. This usually causes only a partial and temporary hearing loss, as the hearing returns to normal when the fluid disperses.

Other problems can affect the middle ear, such as a perforation (hole) of the eardrum, problems with the ossicles, which may be missing, fused together or abnormal. If the child's problem is only a middle ear problem, any hearing loss is usually no more than moderate.

Again, surgery can sometimes help. Most people have come across the 'grommet', a small 'valve' placed across the eardrum to keep the middle ear dry and free of fluid if a child suffers from glue ear. Other surgery, such as patching a perforation of an eardrum, is also possible.

The inner ear

Problems with the inner ear are much less common, but when they do occur, they can cause anything from mild to occasionally total hearing loss. Furthermore, the loss is usually permanent. Inner ear problems usually affect hearing because the sound-sensitive hair cells in the cochlea do not function properly. They may be damaged; they may not have formed properly; they may be totally absent. The cochlea itself may be absent or malformed. The degree of hearing loss is closely related to the state of the hair cells.

Nerve and brain

Conditions that affect the nerve of hearing and the brain do not necessarily affect the cochlea. In other words, they do not affect the child's ability to hear sound. They may, however, affect the child's ability to make sense of that sound. This is an important distinction. It is important to establish whether a child is not hearing sounds properly or just not understanding them properly. If the child is not hearing them properly (because of damage to the cochlea), a hearing aid trial and support aimed at overcoming the deafness are appropriate. If a child is hearing properly but not processing what is heard (i.e. there are problems with the nerve or brain), a hearing aid is not appropriate, and habilitation may be more appropriate from specialists in learning disabilities than from specialists in hearing impairment.

This section has provided a brief overview of the anatomy, physiology and pathology of the hearing system. It has also hopefully equipped the reader better to understand the task of the clinician. He must decide whether there is a problem, how serious it is, what is its nature and cause, and what can be done about it. All this information must be extracted from a frequently moving target who is far too young and far too interested in wreaking havoc with the play dough to be able to answer questions or sit still for half an hour while his ears are tested on a computer. A colleague of mine once began a presentation by saying, 'Paediatric audiology is difficult.' I often think of that remark: it is simple but profound!

How we measure hearing – psychoacoustics

To understand how we measure hearing, it is first necessary to make sure that both parent and professional know what is meant by the words we use. One of the problems with understanding hearing and deafness is that hearing is a common part of life, so is accompanied by a whole range of words commonly used to describe the experience: loud, soft, high, low, mellow, sharp, treble, base, boomy, pitch, frequency, loudness, intensity.... Furthermore, very different words can be used by different people to describe the same sound – think of the variety of words used to describe 'rock' music, often very different depending on whether uttered by parent or teenage child. Some of the terms we will use have strict definitions when used clinically but not when used generally.

Pitch

If you play the notes on a piano starting at the 'bottom' of the keyboard, you will be playing notes that go from low pitch to high pitch. The sound of a bass drum is made up of low-pitched sounds. The sound of a bat's cry is made up of very high-pitched sounds. The sound of the wind is made up of a broad range of low, middle and high pitch sounds mixed together. The world is full of ever-changing sound and combinations of sounds. All the sounds that we hear are made up of combinations of basic sound 'colours' or pitches. The different pitches give the sound its character: higher pitches tend to make sounds 'sharper' or 'brighter'; lower pitches tend to make sounds 'fuller' or more 'mellow'.

Speech is an ever-changing mixture of different pitches. For example, an 'mm' sound is made up of only low pitches. An 'oo' sound is made up of only middle pitches. An 'ss' sound is made up of high pitches. To hear the word 'moose', the ear must be able to pick up the low, then middle, then high pitch sounds in quick succession. Many speech sounds are a mixture of pitches. When listening to everyday conversation, the ear is filtering and analysing a wide range of rapidly changing pitches.

Loudness

Sound is sometimes very loud, such as at a disco. Sometimes, it is so quiet we can hardly hear it, such as when listening for the sound of an animal creeping through the forest. Loudness changes completely independently from pitch. We can have loud, low-pitched sounds (e.g. from a drum struck hard) or quiet, low-pitched sounds (e.g. a drum struck softly). We can have loud, high-pitched sounds (e.g. the screech of a braking bus). We can also have quiet, high-pitched sounds (e.g. the squeak of a mouse).

When listening to music, the ear must cope with a range of loudness, from very soft to very loud. Speech also changes in loudness, and the ear has to cope with rapid changes in loudness when listening to conversation.

Pitch versus loudness

The confusion between pitch and loudness causes one common misunderstanding about partial hearing loss. Some children have what is known as a high pitch hearing loss. They can hear low-pitched sounds well, but not high-pitched ones. They may hear the low-pitched sound of a drum but not the high-pitched squeal of a braking bus. When someone with this loss listens to speech, it will sound perfectly loud enough because they are hearing low pitches normally. However, instead of sounding like normal speech, it will sound muffled because the high pitches are missing. You can get an idea of what this means by covering your mouth with your hand and then talking out loud. Covering your mouth has the effect of taking out the high-pitched sounds. The sound you make will still be (just about) as loud as normal speech. Indeed, you can shout and make it very loud. However, it will not sound normal, or even intelligible, because of the missing high-pitched sounds.

> *Clinician*: 'I'm sure Susie can hear low-pitched sounds.'
> *Parent*: 'I agree. I asked her yesterday if she wanted a sweet. I was only whispering, but she still heard me.'

In the above conversation between a clinician and a parent, the clinician is talking about the pitch of sound that the child can hear, whereas the parent is talking about the loudness of the sound.

Frequency

The term 'frequency' is similar in meaning to the term 'pitch', although in audiology it actually means something very specific.

Sound is caused by vibration. You can see a guitar string vibrate. You can feel a drum skin vibrate. The faster the vibration, the higher in pitch a sound will be. The 'bass' strings on a piano vibrate more slowly than the treble strings. Men's voice boxes vibrate (a little) more slowly than women's do, giving them more bass-sounding voices. The word 'frequency' is used to describe the speed of the vibration that causes the sound. It uses a unit called the hertz (or Hz for short). Hertz are to frequency what metres are to length. One vibration (i.e. one 'in-and-out') every second is referred to as 1 Hz. As the vibration gets faster, so the frequency increases. The human ear can respond to vibrations of between 20 and 20 000 Hz (which goes to show what an extraordinary machine the human ear is – don't even try to imagine an eardrum vibrating that fast!). Most speech sounds occur between 250 and 8000 Hz. It should be noted that these higher-frequency sounds are sometimes referred to in kilohertz or kHz, so that 1000 Hz is 1 kHz, 8000 Hz is 8 kHz and so on.

Strictly speaking, the difference between frequency and pitch is that 'frequency' describes the vibrations themselves, whilst 'pitch' describes our experience of the vibration and may vary from person to person.

Intensity

The word 'intensity' is used to describe the size of the vibration that causes the sound. It uses a unit called the decibel (or dB for short). Decibels are to intensity what minutes are to time. As the vibration gets bigger, so the intensity increases. The human ear can respond to intensities of between 0 and 100 dB. Sounds that are more intense than 100 dB tend to sound uncomfortably loud (Figure 1.2).

Strictly speaking then, the difference between intensity and loudness is that 'intensity' describes the vibrations themselves, whereas 'loudness' describes our experience of the vibrations. The difference becomes clear when we compare the experience of someone with normal hearing and someone with severe hearing loss. If they both listen to a sound with an *intensity* of 90 dB, what they hear will be quite different. To one, the sound will be very *loud*; to the other it may be very *quiet*.

The audiogram – measuring frequency and intensity

The audiogram has a central place in hearing measurement. Indeed, there is some concern that it can be given too much emphasis. It is certainly a useful summary of how much a child can hear, and a significant part of early hearing assessment is aimed at building up a clear picture of the audiogram.

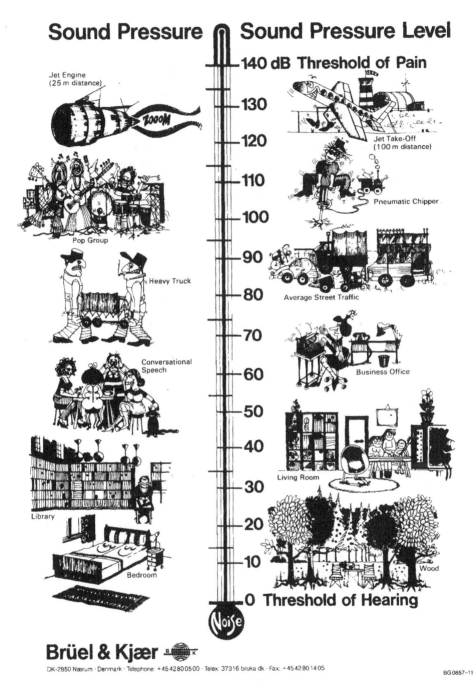

Figure 1.2 Scale showing the intensity of different sounds in decibels (dB). Reproduced by kind permission of Brüel & Kjær.

When hearing is tested, one object of the test is to find out which frequencies the ear can respond to. The most common frequencies tested are those which make up speech. These are from around 250 to around 8000 Hz. Typically, the frequencies are laid out along the top of an audiogram as follows:

250   500   1000   2000   4000   8000   Hz

When we test hearing, we are trying to measure the intensity a sound must reach before the ear can detect it. This point at which the sound is just detected is called the 'threshold'. People with normal hearing have thresholds of around 0 dB for each frequency. Someone with a severe hearing loss may have a threshold of around 80 dB.

Intensity is laid along the side of the audiogram as follows:

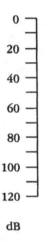

Combining the frequency and intensity scales gives the full audiogram:

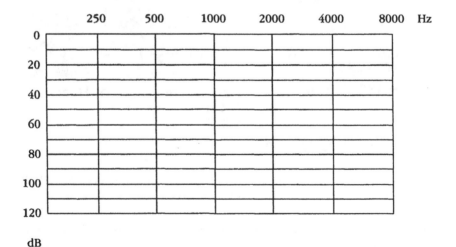

For older, co-operative children, it is usually a straightforward exercise to find out how well they can hear. Sounds of different frequency are played to them, one ear at a time, through headphones, and the intensity needed to just hear each sound is recorded.

The British Association of Teachers of the Deaf (BATOD) (British Society of Audiology, 1988) has put forward definitions of the degree of hearing loss. The terms it uses have come into common usage in audiology. BATOD talks about normal, mild, moderate, severe and profound hearing loss, intending the words to describe a gradual change from one to the other. They are described as in Table 1.1.

Table 1.1.

Degree of hearing loss	Hearing level in dB
Normal	0–19
Mild	20–40
Moderate	41–70
Severe	71–95
Profound	95+

'Average hearing loss' means the average of the thresholds between 250 and 4000 Hz.

In the author's experience, these terms can cast as much confusion and darkness as light unless used very carefully. The problem is that the words can give a false impression of the level of difficulty the child will face. The numbers in Table 1.1 imply that the difference between, for example, moderate and severe hearing loss is not all that great. However, the difference between the images conjured up by the terms 'moderate' (which can imply not too bad) and 'severe' (which can imply catastrophic) may be a yawning gulf.

It is worth looking at some examples of typical audiograms in order to get a feel for what they mean.

Normal hearing

Figure 1.3 shows an example of normal hearing. The circles represent the intensity at which the sound can just be heard at each frequency. All the circles are on or close to 0 dB. Hearing is therefore normal.

High-frequency hearing loss

Figure 1.4 shows an example of a hearing loss for high frequencies. The circles are at 0 dB for low-frequency sounds but at 70 dB for high-frequency sounds. This child has a high-frequency hearing loss, so will

AUDIOGRAM

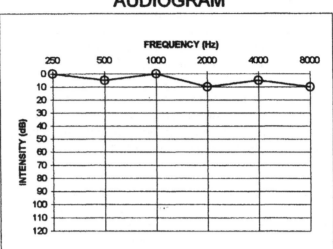

Figure 1.3 Audiogram showing normal hearing. The circles at each frequency are above the 10 dB line.

not hear the high-frequency sounds of speech unless they are amplified. However, he will hear the low-frequency sounds normally. The child will need a hearing aid that amplifies only the high frequencies.

Severe hearing loss

Figure 1.5 shows an example of severe hearing loss. For this child, no sound can be heard until the intensities are raised to around 80 dB. This is a severe loss, and the child will need hearing aids to amplify all the different frequencies.

Profound hearing loss

Figure 1.6 shows an example of a child with a profound loss. This child can only detect a few low-frequency sounds. Even these can only be detected if the intensity is 90 dB or more. He cannot hear the high-frequency sounds at all. This child will need powerful hearing aids but will still not hear high frequencies.

One important point about the audiogram is that it tells us not only the severity of the hearing loss, but also which sounds a hearing aid must amplify most. There is a very wide range of hearing aids available, and the clinician carefully tests the hearing in part so that he can select the right hearing aid for the child. This topic will be returned to in Chapter 3.

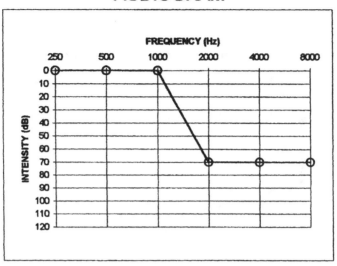

Figure 1.4 High-frequency hearing loss. The circles are at 0 db for low frequencies (250–1000 Hz) but at 70 dB for high frequencies (2000–8000 dB).

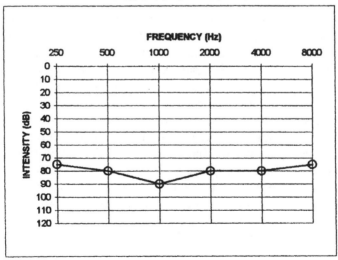

Figure 1.5 All the circles are around the 80 dB level.

AUDIOGRAM

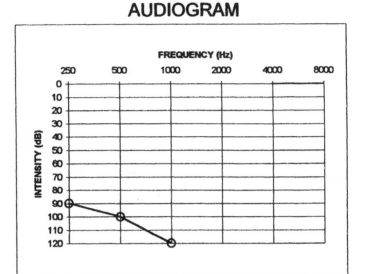

Figure 1.6 Profound hearing loss. The only responses are to low frequency (250–1000 Hz). The child does not hear higher-frequency sounds at all.

This section has described the audiogram as a chart on which frequency and intensity are plotted. This chart is used to record the state of the child's hearing and to help us to select the right hearing aid when necessary.

How do they know he's deaf? – testing hearing

The clinician has a number of measurement tools at his disposal. Parents will find their child being put through a variety of different hearing tests. It is useful for them to understand what is involved with each kind of test, the reason for doing that particular test and what kind of information it gives. There are no standard models for assessing hearing loss in the UK or the USA. Some clinics are extremely well equipped and organized. Others are much more primitive. Hearing is a critical sense, and parents have the right to make sure that their child receives sufficiently thorough investigation. For that reason also, they need to know what tests are possible and to explore with their own service what is appropriate and what is not appropriate in the case of their own child.

The next section looks at ways in which hearing can be measured. The aim is to explain what tests can be carried out, how they work, what information they give and when it is appropriate to use them.

The general purpose of most hearing tests is to provide information to 'fill in' the audiogram, in other words to establish what frequencies and at what intensities a child can hear. Another important set of tests looks at the way in which the child uses his hearing in everyday life.

Hearing Tests

Children are never too young to be tested. Hearing tests now exist that can measure the hearing of babies as soon as they are born. It is no longer necessary to put off testing hearing until the baby is 'old enough to co-operate'.

There are two kinds of hearing test: behavioural tests and objective tests. Behavioural tests require the child to respond in some way to a sound. For example, asking a child to put a man in a boat when he hears the sound is a behavioural test. Objective tests do not require a child to respond. For example, putting a probe in the child's ear and measuring the echo that comes back from the cochlea does not require the child to do anything (except sit still!). This is an objective test. The advantage of behavioural tests, for children who can do them, is usually that they provide more comprehensive and more accurate information. The advantage of objective tests is that, for children who are too young or too developmentally delayed to co-operate with behavioural tests, information about their hearing can still be obtained. Below, we will look at both types of test. Objective tests are described first as these are often the tests first encountered.

Objective tests

The main virtue of objective tests is that they give us a measure of hearing without any active co-operation from the child. The tests do require the child to be still, however, and achieving that requirement alone can make for interesting times in an audiology department.

Otoacoustic emissions

If a click sound is played directly into the ear canal of a normal ear, the cochlea will generate a small echo. If an echo is normal, we can say that the hearing system from the outer ear to the cochlea is working well. We cannot comment about the system beyond the cochlea, but we can say that, because the emission is normal, the cochlea is normal and the child does not need a hearing aid and aural habilitation. That finding can be a major step in a child's investigation.

If there is no echo, we are in a much weaker position. All we can say is that this child might have a hearing problem. In fact, even some children with normal hearing have no echo. Therefore, all we can really say about a child with no echo is that he needs further investigation.

The test is known as an otoacoustic emissions (OAE) test. The equipment for carrying out the test consists of a small probe attached to a special computer, which generates the click and measures the echo.

The probe is placed gently into the child's ear, and a series of clicks is presented to the ear. During this time, the child must remain still. It is best, although not essential, if he is asleep. If the child does move, however, the computer can detect this and temporarily stop recording. When a clear picture of the ear's response has been built up, the machine stops automatically.

Sample results from an OAE test are shown in Figures 1.7 and 1.8.

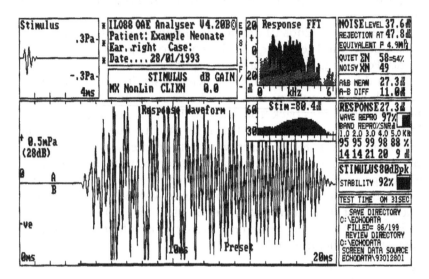

Figure 1.7 Otoacoustic emission. This test report shows a normal emission. It looks complicated, but the important section is the box marked 'Response FFT'. A black 'mountain range' can be seen above grey 'foothills'. The black area shows the echo, or emission from the cochlea. This emission is only seen in a healthy cochlea.

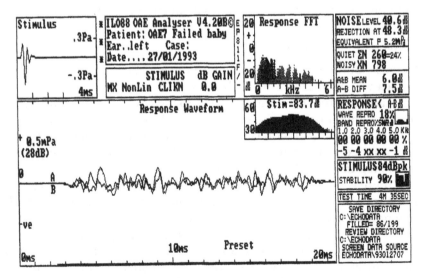

Figure 1.8 The absence of otoacoustic emission. In this test report, the black 'mountain range' is not present. However, all this result tells us is that the hearing *may* not be normal, so it should be investigated further. Even mild losses can eliminate the emission, and emissions can be absent even though the hearing is normal.

Evoked response testing

When a sound enters the cochlea, the cochlea changes that sound from a mechanical vibration to a nerve impulse. This nerve impulse then travels up the nerve of hearing, through the brainstem and into the brain. As it makes this journey, it passes through several different relay stations on the way. Evoked response testing is a way of following the nerve impulse's journey through these various relay stations.

We can follow the journey all the way from the cochlea to the brain, getting different responses from different relay stations *en route*. However, the most useful response is one that comes from the brainstem and is known, rather unexcitingly, as wave V. The wave V response is closely related to the threshold for hearing. In other words, the intensity at which we start to see the response is also the intensity at which the child will start to hear the sound. When we are testing for it, the test is usually known as auditory brainstem response (ABR) testing.

The test both tells us whether the child has a problem and gives us some idea of the severity of that problem. The intensity at which we get the response has been shown to be closely related to the high-frequency hearing. If we get an ABR threshold of 80 dB, we can say that the child's hearing for high-frequency sounds will be close to 80 dB. It does not tell us anything about the low frequencies. (Work is currently under way to enable us to use the ABR test to look at low-frequency hearing, but this is much more difficult, and clinicians vary in their faith in the methods that have been tried; see Baldwin and Watkin, 1997, for a discussion.)

If we get no response on ABR testing, this means that the high-frequency hearing thresholds are worse than the limits to which the equipment will test. Many ABR systems only test to 90 dB. A lack of response with such a system does not necessarily mean that the child has no high-frequency hearing, only that the hearing is poorer than 90 dB.

The test needs between 30 minutes and an hour to complete, and the child needs to be asleep (although you can test an awake child as long as he is still). The test involves attaching electrodes (sticky pads that conduct electricity) to the forehead and behind each ear. These are then connected to a special computer (Figure 1.9). The computer picks up the nerve impulses through the electrodes. A headphone is then held gently against the ear, and click sounds are played at different levels. The test aims to establish whether there is a wave V response and, if so, the quietest level at which it can be detected.

The ABR test can be carried out in more or less any quiet place. It is sometimes carried out in the audiology department. When children are older and may not settle easily, it is possible to give them sedation. If a child also needs an ear examination under anaesthetic, and possibly ear surgery (such as grommet insertion), the ABR test can be performed in the operating theatre. It is occasionally performed at home, with the child asleep in his own bed.

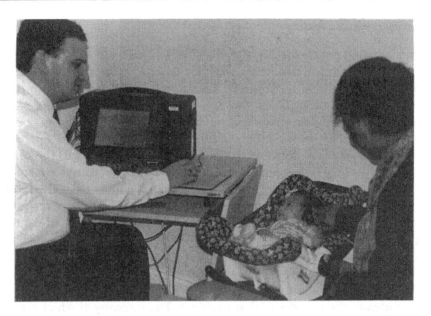

Figure 1.9 Auditory brainstem response testing. The baby has three electrodes stuck to the skin, usually one on the forehead and one behind each ear. The mother is holding a headphone against the baby's left ear while the technician runs the test.

Other forms of evoked response testing may occasionally be encountered. It is possible to follow the nerve impulses all the way from the cochlea to the brain itself. In practice, there are problems in trying to do this with young children. The cochlea response is very tiny and can often only be recorded clearly by using a special needle, which has to be inserted through the drum. This test is called electrocochleography, and, although it is used, it is not common. Responses at the higher brain centres can only be recorded from patients who are awake and still (a contradiction in terms for anyone under 3 years old!) for about an hour, so they are not really used on young children.

Figures 1.10 and 1.11 show examples of traces from an ABR test.

Impedance testing

This test measures the stiffness, or impedance, of the eardrum under different conditions of pressure. In its main form, it is used not to test hearing but to check whether the middle ear is performing normally. This is particularly useful with children, who are very prone to the problem of glue ear.

The test works by producing very slight movements of the eardrum and measuring whether these movements are normal. The movements are produced by holding a mushroom-shaped probe gently against the ear and producing small pressure changes between the probe and the eardrum. These pressure changes should move the eardrum in and

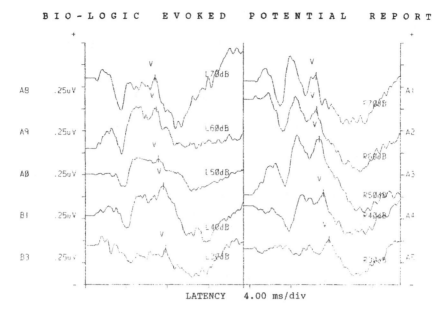

Figure 1.10 A normal auditory brainstem response result. The waves represent the response of the ear and brain to sounds played through the headphones. The important wave is wave V, which has been marked. This wave can be clearly seen in the left and right ears even when the sounds are at a low intensity of 30 dB. This result tells us that the hearing in this frequency region (2–4 kHz) is better than 30 dB.

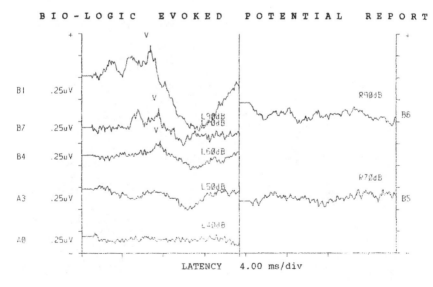

Figure 1.11 An abnormal auditory brainstem response. The left ear shows a wave V at 60 dB and possibly at 50 dB, but not at 40 dB. In the right ear, there is no wave V, even at 90 dB. This result tells us that the high-frequency hearing is below normal in both ears, but worse in the right ear, where the high-frequency threshold is poorer than 90 dB.

out. As the drum moves, it stiffens. The amount of stiffness is measured by bouncing a sound off the eardrum at the same time and measuring how much sound is reflected back. The test takes only a few seconds, although again it requires the child to be reasonably still (Figure 1.12).

The change in stiffness is plotted on a chart called a tympanogram. There are three common types of tympanogram, each associated with different states of the middle ear. Figure 1.13 shows various tympanogram types.

Figure 1.13a shows a normal tympanogram in each ear, a 'mountain' with its peak on the zero of the pressure scale. This means that the eardrum is mobile and that its greatest mobility is at atmospheric pressure (represented by the zero on the scale).

In Figure 1.13b, the peaks of the tympanograms are shifted to the left. This means that there is slight negative pressure behind each eardrum, a common effect of a cold.

In Figure 1.13c, the tympanogram traces are flat. This result is typical of a child with fluid behind the eardrums, such as in glue ear. Note that the exact interpretation of a flat trace needs care as other conditions can also give a similar trace. The interpretation is made by looking at both the shape of the trace and various other measures that are printed out with it.

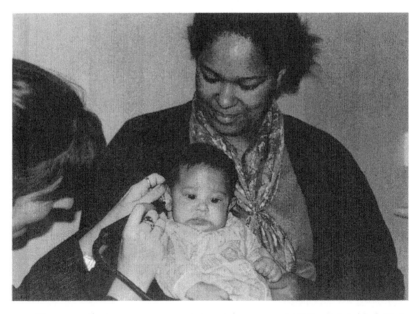

Figure 1.12 Impedance testing. A small probe is gently placed in the child's ear. The test causes a pressure change in the ear (no worse than being under 20 cm of bath water), which changes the stiffness of the eardrum. This change in stiffness is measured by reflecting sound off the eardrum while the pressure is changing.

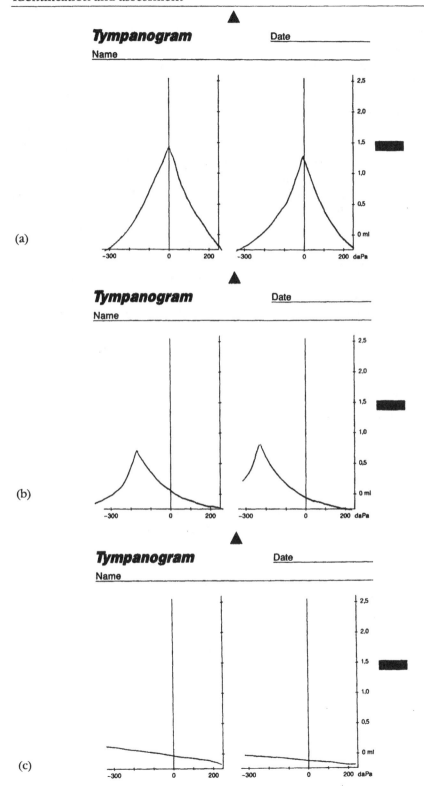

Figure 1.13 Results from impedance testing. See the text for an explanation.

Impedance is a very different type of test from the ABR and OAE tests. It is also a much misunderstood test. It is important to remember that the tympanogram only shows the state of the middle ear. It is not a hearing test. A normal tympanogram does not mean normal hearing. A child can have a profound hearing loss as a result of cochlea damage and still have a perfectly normal middle ear. In the same way, checking the tyre pressures on a car will not tell you whether the engine is working.

There is a way in which the impedance test can be used to give some idea of the hearing. This is called stapedius reflex testing. It relies on the fact that there is a small muscle in the middle ear, called the stapedius muscle, which tightens and stiffens the eardrum when a loud sound is heard. The muscle only tightens if the sound is loud to the listener. This tightening changes the stiffness of the eardrum, which can be detected by the impedance meter. The test works by playing a loud sound through the probe and looking for any change in the stiffness of the drum. If the change does occur, we know that the child is hearing the sound and that it is loud to him.

A profoundly deaf child, for example, will not hear the sound, so the muscle will not tighten. Unfortunately, the relationship between the reflex threshold (i.e. the level that just triggers the reflex) and the hearing threshold is not very close. It is possible to have quite severe cochlear damage and still produce a reflex. Also, any middle ear condition (and even a grommet) stops us being able to measure the reflex. These limitations mean that the reflex threshold can serve only as a rough guide to the underlying level of hearing.

Behavioural tests

Behavioural tests require the tester to tease out from the child some response to sound that can be seen and preferably repeated. In many cases, the success of our efforts is entirely dependent on winning over the child and getting him to perform with us. Children are not always willing to fall in with our plans. If we are to test a child successfully, we may need to let him thaw out slowly, take time to get to know him and give him an element of control so that he feels less intimidated. A hearing test is a test on a part of the child that does not work well. We are making life deliberately difficult for him. Maybe he doesn't always want to co-operate, do well, perform, try. Perhaps we should all have a hearing test to remind us how hard it is and that he's only a little kid who should be playing in the park.

Behavioural observation audiometry

This is the earliest behavioural test that can be used on a child. Before around 6 months of age, children do not have good control over their own responses to sound. Responses between birth and 6 months tend to be reflex responses, such as startling to a loud sound, stilling to an interesting sound, stirring or opening the eyes wide to a novel sound, changing the sucking pattern when a new sound is introduced, or even waking from sleep to a sound. Typically in behavioural observation audiometry (BOA), a child is observed closely while lying comfortably on a mat, in a bouncer or on a parent's lap (Figure 1.14). Sounds are periodically presented and a response looked for. The intensity of the sound that produced the response is recorded. Low, middle or high frequency sounds can be used.

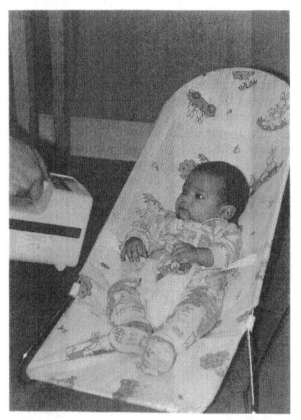

Figure 1.14 Behavioural observation audiometry. The tester presents a sound through a hand-held sound generator. In this case, the baby has responded with eye-widening and hand movement.

There are many problems with BOA. Unless complex and time-consuming procedures are used, it is difficult to get clear, repeatable responses. Also, the clinician has to decide whether a response is present or absent, and this is a notoriously difficult thing to do, leaving much to the clinician's skill at reading children. Studies (see Wilson and Thompson, 1984, for a review) have shown BOA to be an unreliable tool and to give at best a crude measure of hearing. The author has found it most effective in looking at a child's responses while asleep. These responses vary. Examples are altered breathing rate, stirring, blinking, sucking and waking. The responses are often clear and can help at least to tell the difference between hearing and no hearing at different frequencies. It would, however, be very rare today to find clinicians relying solely on BOA.

Distraction testing

When children reach a developmental age of around 6 months, they will begin to look for the source of a sound. This behaviour is used in the distraction method (Ewing and Ewing, 1944; McCormick, 1993) to give a more accurate picture of a child's hearing. In this technique, the child sits on a parent's knee. One tester distracts the child in front, while the other presents sounds from behind. If the child hears the sound, he will usually turn to locate it (Figure 1.15). This method can be used to check the child's responses to a range of frequencies and to check each ear separately. In experienced hands, it can be a useful test. However, it is fraught with pitfalls. In particular, if not carefully carried out, it can lead to even profoundly deaf children 'passing' the test. Deaf children are very visual and may catch sight of the tester out of the corner of their eye. They may see a shadow as the tester moves to present the sound. They may smell perfume as the tester gets ready to apply the test. They may feel the movement of air as the tester makes speech sounds from close behind them.

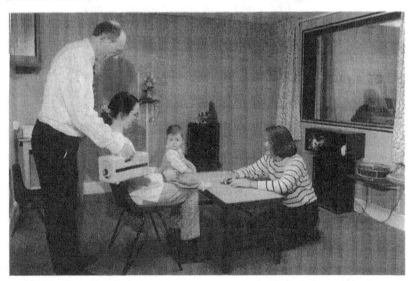

Figure 1.15 Distraction testing. The child is distracted by one tester, while the other presents noises from behind. This picture shows the child turning to look for the source of the sound.

Distraction testing is most successful between 6 months and 2 years of age.

Visual reinforcement audiometry

Visual reinforcement audiometry (VRA) is another test that works well from 6 months of age, although it can also be useful for much older children who have proved difficult to test by other means. This test involves presenting sounds from one side of the child. When the child turns to look, he is presented with a visual reward such as a teddy bear with eyes flashing, a dancing pig or a whirling 'ambulance' light. The child quickly learns to associate the sound and the reward. Many children find the 'game' fascinating, and, by a judicious use of different visual rewards, they can be kept going for a long time while a range of information is obtained.

When sounds are presented through loudspeakers, it is difficult to separate out differences between ears as the sound will be detected by whichever ear works best. One way around this is to check the child's ability to pinpoint where sounds are coming from. The child is called first from one loudspeaker and then from the other. If both ears are hearing equally well, the child should look quickly at whichever speaker the voice is coming from.

Performance testing

From two and a half years onwards, many children will be able to carry out performance testing. In such tests, they have to perform a simple task whenever they hear a sound. A wide variety of games can be drawn upon to keep the child performing while information is obtained. However, the most common game when this test is first encountered is the ubiquitous man-in-the-boat game. In this game, a child is trained to put a man in a boat when they hear a sound. It can take quite a long time for young children to carry this out reliably. Training is best done by showing the child what to do, rather than by explaining it to him. In the hands of an experienced clinician, the test is a good one, but it may take some time to convince parents that the child's actions are genuine responses to sound rather than lucky guesses, flukes, random play or generally having a good time!

Sounds for this game can be presented through loudspeakers (the test then commonly being known as a 'free-field' test) or through headphones. If headphones are used, accurate information can be obtained about each ear separately.

A recent innovation is the use of insert-phones. These are small inserts, with soft foam tips, that are pushed gently into the ear canal. Young children often find them more acceptable than headphones, and they can be used to get information about each ear separately on both performance testing and VRA.

If a child is suffering conductive hearing loss because of middle ear problems, it is sometimes useful to know how well the inner ear is working. This is particularly true for children with bilateral atresia, when the problem will be with them for many years. To measure inner ear function, the VRA test can be conducted, while the sound is presented through a small vibrator placed behind the ear and held in place by a headband. This is called bone conduction testing. The vibrator, or bone conductor as it is called, stimulates the bones of the head. This allows the sound to be fed directly into the inner ear. The sounds are not affected by any blockage of the middle or outer ear. The hearing of the inner ear can then be measured.

Interpreting results

Results for all of the tests described above can be transferred onto an audiogram chart, and it should be routine practice for the clinician to go through the results on the chart with parents at the end of each testing session. Testing can be carried out with and without hearing aids. Some of the symbols used on the audiogram are standard, in particular an 'O' for the right ear tested under headphones, and an 'X' for the left. Other symbols vary from clinic to clinic.

It is useful to have a look at examples of different audiograms and their interpretation.

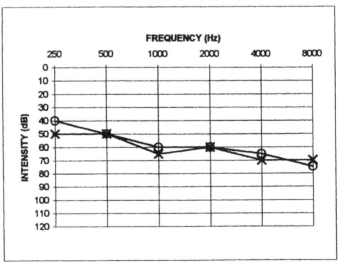

Figure 1.16 Bilateral moderate hearing loss. ○ = right ear; ✕ = left ear.

AUDIOGRAM

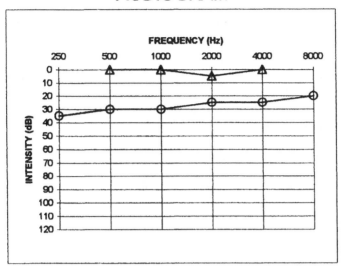

Figure 1.17 Mild conductive hearing loss. This is a typical result for a child with glue ear. ○ = right ear; △ = bone conduction.

Figure 1.16 shows the results for a child with a similar hearing loss in both ears when tested through headphones.

Figure 1.17 shows a child with a mild loss in his right ear when tested through headphones but normal hearing when tested with the bone

AUDIOGRAM

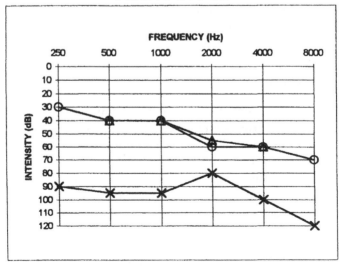

Figure 1.18 Audiogram showing mild sensorineural hearing loss in the right ear and severe hearing loss in the left. ○ = right ear; ✕ = left ear; △ = bone conduction.

conductor. This child has a conductive loss, which is typical of a child with glue ear.

Figure 1.18 shows a child with a moderate loss in the right ear and a severe loss in the left. The bone conduction responses suggest that the loss is sensorineural rather than conductive (although interpreting bone conduction can be quite difficult when the ears are not the same).

Figure 1.19 shows a young child tested through loudspeakers with and without hearing aids. It is possible to see the improvement in hearing that the aids can give.

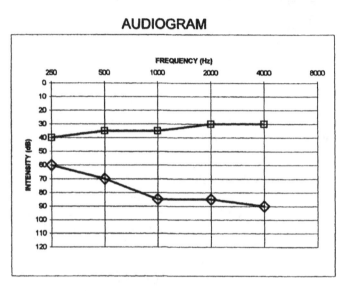

Figure 1.19 Free-field (loudspeaker) audiogram with and without hearing aids. ◇ = free-field unaided; □ = free-field aided.

Speech discrimination testing

A child's ability to understand speech is all important. Speech tests can be used from as early as a child can begin to perform reliable behavioural testing, and the results can make more sense to parents than all the other whistles and squawks that are used. However, in the early stages, speech testing is given less emphasis. This is because a knowledge of hearing for specific frequencies is more important in helping us to assess the degree and cause of the loss and in selecting hearing aids. The first 'speech' testing is typically carried out by seeing at what intensities a child responds to typical speech sounds. The Ling sounds ('mm', 'oo', 'ee', 'ah', 'sh' and 'ss') are commonly used as these sounds span the frequency range.

As a child gets older, other formal speech tests can be used. One common test is the McCormick Toy Test (McCormick, 1993), in which a child points to one toy out of several placed in front of him. The toys form pairs, each pair sounding similar (cup and duck, tree and key, etc.), and the tester measures the intensity at which the child can point to them accurately. This test can be done with and without lip-reading. Other tests may involve repeating words or sentences, pointing at pictures and so on. Background noise is sometimes used to make the test more 'realistic'.

No test is an island, entire unto itself

In the pursuit of a clear picture of a child's hearing, no single test alone will suffice. Because children, particularly very young children, can be very difficult to test accurately, it is useful to combine information from several different tests to see whether they are providing compatible or contradictory results. Additionally, some tests only give at best partial information, and a range of tests may be needed to give the full picture.

The following case studies illustrate the use of tests in combination and the gradual building up of a picture of the hearing loss.

Case study

John was seen for assessment as a baby. He had had a stormy time as a neonate. His parents felt that there was something not right with his hearing but that he clearly responded by jumping to loud noises. He was tested first with OAE. This showed no clear echo, establishing that he was a child who needed further investigation.

John was tested with ABR in the audiology unit. There was no measurable response, suggesting that his high-frequency hearing was worse than 90 dB (the limit to which the equipment will test). Impedance testing showed normal tympanograms, which suggested that the middle ears were not congested. He was tested with BOA, but the only response was a possible stilling response to a loud 'Boo!'.

The results clearly showed that John had a hearing problem. We used the results to plot an audiogram as best we could. His high frequencies were poorer than 90 dB, and there was possibly some low-frequency hearing, as suggested from his behavioural response. The audiogram is shown in Figure 1.20.

John was fitted with hearing aids at 2 months of age.

When John was 4 months old, a home visit was made to repeat objective testing because John was becoming too old for us to be able to guarantee that he would sleep if we tested him in the clinic. There was still no response on ABR testing to 90 dB. There was again no echo on OAE. Impedance testing showed normal tympanometry, suggesting that the

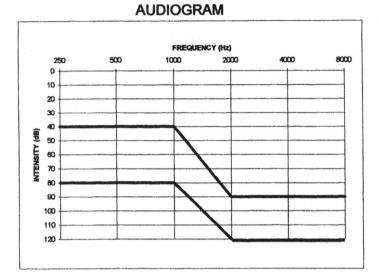

Figure 1.20 Estimated area of hearing for John (see text).

loss was not conductive. BOA was carried out, the intention being to see whether John could be woken from sleep. The results were interesting. A low-frequency (500 Hz) noise of 75 dB did not wake him, but he did start sucking furiously in his sleep. This response was repeatable. He did the same with an 1000 Hz noise at 90 dB. Again, this was repeatable. John did not respond to any sound at higher frequencies. Clearly, he was hearing low-frequency sounds but not high-frequency ones. These results suggested that our audiogram was a reasonable estimate.

By 11 months of age (or 6 months developmentally), John was testable using VRA, and we obtained the thresholds shown in Figure 1.21. Using insert-phones, we were able to test left and right ears separately.

At 14 months old, John was tested with VRA, and his thresholds seemed to have worsened by a further 20 dB. Impedance testing on this occasion showed flat tympanograms. John was seen by the ENT consultant, who diagnosed fluid behind the eardrum. This cleared after 2 months, at which time his hearing returned to where it had been before the middle ear fluid appeared. The tympanograms were also normal again.

This section has given 'thumbnail' sketches of many of the tests of hearing in children. All of these should be available as they can all, in their own way, provide pieces of the puzzle and help us to build a true picture of the hearing as early as possible.

AUDIOGRAM

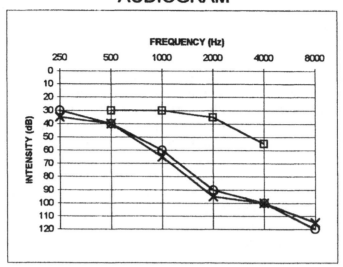

Figure 1.21 John's hearing when tested with insert phones and then with hearing aids. O = right ear (insert phone); X = left ear (insert phone); □ = aided.

How soon can deafness be detected – child surveillance for hearing

Some parents of hearing impaired children have great concerns that the hearing loss was not picked up earlier. They sometimes blame themselves for failing to notice tell-tale signs. They sometimes blame their local service for not checking the child 'properly'. For children who do not develop reasonable speech, language and communication with hearing aids, the question 'Would he have done better if he had been detected earlier?' may never really go away.

In reality, hearing loss can be very difficult to detect. If the loss is mild, the child may cope well enough (respond to sound, albeit a bit sluggishly; start talking, although perhaps delayed and not clear). Even children with profound losses can remain undetected for a surprisingly long time. They develop almost supersensitive vision and can use this so cleverly that they detect things of which we are not aware. When they are called from behind, they may turn and so appear to hear, when in fact they have caught sight of a shadow or a reflection in the window, or even smelt the faint tang of perfume.

The early detection of hearing loss is partly a question of organization. In order for hearing loss to be discovered, there needs to be a programme of systematic searching across all children in a district. Such a programme is referred to as a child surveillance programme for hearing. It relies on finding effective ways of 'screening' all children. Screening means giving a simple but sensitive test that normal hearing children will pass and hearing impaired children will fail. The organization of child surveillance programmes (and wider aspects of the audiology services) in the UK has in the past been variable and in some places quite idiosyncratic. Until recently, no clear guidelines for such services existed.

There has increasingly been recognition that children detected early have a better chance of developing speech and language than children detected late. This is probably more true for children with more severe hearing losses. Following concern that children were not being picked up early enough, the National Deaf Children's Society (NDCS; 1994, 1996) has recently published a set of Quality Standards in Paediatric Audiology. These publications deal with both the detection of hearing impaired children and the habilitation of children identified as having hearing loss. They set targets for services and describe the key factors of a service that will enable those targets to be met.

The NDCS targets are:

- to detect 80% of bilateral congenital hearing impairment in excess of 50 dB HL (averaged across 500, 1000, 2000 and 4000 Hz) within the first year of life, and 40% by the age of 6 months
- to fit hearing aids within 4 weeks of confirmation of hearing loss
- to test children at high risk of acquired loss (e.g. following meningitis) within 4 weeks of referral
- to ensure that by 1 year of age, all children have a formal hearing screen or surveillance procedure.

The health services have found these targets challenging, to say the least. The first, in particular, is driven by the need to bring age of detection down. Many districts have in the past detected hearing loss through a child surveillance programme that was a combination of health visitor distraction testing and relying on parental or professional (health visitor, GP, etc.) concern. A number of health districts (see for example, Shiu et al., 1996) have measured how well their programmes perform, and the answer has been 'not well'. Typically, over 50% of children are not identified until they are at least 1 year old.

More recently, two models for child surveillance programmes have been suggested, both of which appear to yield better detection rates.

Model 1

- *Targeted neonatal screening*: Testing at birth all babies who are at risk of deafness (usually all babies who have spent more than 48 hours on the special care baby unit, or where there is a family history of hearing loss, or some other defined risk factor). These babies can be tested with ABR and OAE.

plus

- *Health visitor distraction screening*: Testing all babies at around 8 months of age with a screening version of the distraction test.

Model 2

- *Universal neonatal screening*: Testing at birth all babies in the district. Babies can be tested with ABR and OAE.

There are arguments for and against both models, and the reader is referred to Davis et al. (1997) for a fuller discussion of these arguments. It is clear that whatever system is used, it must be accompanied by high levels of awareness and vigilance on the part of all professionals and of parents, who should receive information about signs of possible hearing loss. One commonly used information sheet is the 'Hints for Parents' sheet shown in Figure 1.22.

It is also clear that any system must also be accompanied by access to a paediatric audiology service of high quality and capable of swift response where concern about a child exists. Each district service should

Hints for Parents

Can your baby hear you?

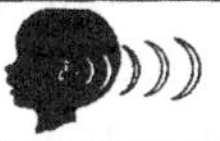

Here is a checklist of some of the general signs you can look for in your baby's first year: YES/NO

Shortly after birth
Your baby should be startled by a sudden loud noise such as a hand clap or a door slamming and should blink or open his eyes widely to such sounds.

By 1 Month
Your baby should be beginning to notice sudden prolonged sounds like the noise of a vacuum cleaner and she should pause and listen to them when they begin.

By 4 Months
He should quieten or smile to the sound of your voice even when he cannot see you. He may also turn his head or eyes toward you if you come up from behind and speak to him from the side.

By 7 Months
She should turn immediately to your voice across the room or to very quiet noises made on each side if she is not too occupied with other things.

By 9 Months
He should listen attentively to familiar everyday sounds and search for very quiet sounds made out of sight. He should also show pleasure in babbling loudly and tunefully.

By 12 Months
She should show some response to her own name and to other familiar words. She may also respond when you say 'no' and 'bye bye' even when she cannot see any accompanying gesture.

> Your health visitor will perform a routine hearing screening test on your baby between six and eight months of age. She will be able to help and advise you at any time before or after this test if you are concerned about your baby and his development. If you suspect that your baby is not hearing normally, either because you cannot answer yes to the items above or for some other reason, then seek advice from your health visitor.

©
Produced by Dr. Barry McCormick
Children's Hearing Assessment Centre, Nottingham
Printed by The Sherwood Press (Nottingham) Limited

Figure 1.22 'Hints for Parents' information sheet. Reproduced by kind permission of B. McCormick.

have a named person who is in charge of the paediatric audiology programme in terms of screening, assessment and habilitation (National Deaf Children's Society, 1996). All staff involved with hearing testing in the district should clearly understand the referral routes into the audiology department. Those involved in screening tests should work to clear and written guidelines. In the guidelines there should be included a 'fast-track' route through to audiology, where there is sufficient concern. Awareness should be promoted by arranging information sessions regularly through the year for health visitors, GPs, paediatricians and all professionals involved in working with children.

Publication of the NDCS Quality Standards has been an influential force for improvement across the UK. The Standards are in the form of two refreshingly slim but still comprehensive booklets, and the reader is recommended to look at them for the clarity and detail that they offer.

In summary, this section has discussed the importance of the early detection of hearing problems and described the different approaches to achieving early detection that exist. It has also discussed the NDCS Quality Standards, which have had a significant influence on the debate on paediatric audiology service provision.

To whom can I turn? – breaking the news

If a child has a significant hearing loss, he needs help. Despite all the processes and systems described above, getting that help can still be a nightmare. Parents tell how, for months, their GP would not believe them; how their child passed (scraped through) the health visitor test although they knew there was a problem; how the audiologists kept bringing him back and back but could not make up their minds; how the ENT consultant set him back a year by assuring them that it was probably just glue ear and would go away by itself in the end; how they became so frustrated that nobody could tell them what had happened, why their child had been singled out to be deaf; how they were moved from doctor to doctor and nobody seemed to know quite what was going on.

The confirmation of hearing loss and subsequent action need careful and sensitive handling. It is important for the clinician to give sufficient time to explain the results to parents, in a place that gives them the privacy to express their grief and ask any questions free from interruption. This should be done in a manner that is sensitive to the parents' reactions.

In some cases, the results will be unequivocal, and the information can be presented with reasonable certainty. In other cases, the results are much less clear cut. Particularly with young children, it can take months to move from identifying that there is a problem, to unveiling the true extent of that problem. This needs to be made clear to the parents, and the clinician needs to be completely open and honest with them, without giving them a false sense of hope but also without undue pessimism when much is still unknown. It is frustrating for parents not to have the whole truth straight away, and it is difficult for them to take in the complexities of just what the tests are and are not telling them. (One of the points of this book is to make that process easier.) Indeed, many are so 'shell-shocked' with the news that they cannot really take in anything beyond that their child is **deaf**.

The clinician may say:

I'm sorry Mr and Mrs Jones, but I am afraid our results show that Anne has a significant hearing loss. In other words, she is a little bit deaf. She can hear some sounds but not others. The cause of this is probably that she was born prematurely and had very high levels of jaundice. The loss is probably not going to get better, and we will need to fit her with some hearing aids. I'm sure if we can get the aids on early, she will do very well, and, because we have discovered the hearing loss in time, she has every chance of developing good speech and language. Do you have any questions for me at this stage?

But what the parent hears is:

I'm sorry Mr and Mrs Jones, but I am afraid our results show that Anne has a significant hearing loss. In other words, she is a little bit deaf. She can hear some sounds but not others. The cause of this is probably that she was born prematurely and had very high levels of jaundice. The loss is probably not going to get better, and we will need to fit her with some hearing aids. I'm sure if we can get the aids on early she will do very well, and, because we have discovered the hearing loss in time, she has every chance of developing good speech and language. Do you have any questions for me at this stage?

The parents should never leave the department without being given the name and telephone number of a clearly defined person whom they can contact with any questions at all and hopefully at any time. The clinician whose responsibility it is to break the news will again vary from district to district. In some cases, it will be an ENT consultant or audiological physician. In others, it may be a senior audiological scientist or community paediatrician. It all depends on how the service is organized in a district.

Although the audiology professionals may vary from district to district, certain processes should always begin once confirmation has been made. Support from an early language adviser/educational audiologist/teacher of the deaf should start as soon as possible. (In some districts, the teaching and support services team is contacted by the audiology department as soon as the parents leave the department. The team usually arranges to visit the home within 24 hours.)

The child will need to see various medical specialists. An ENT consultation will be needed to establish whether the child's condition is treatable medically or surgically. A paediatrician will need to carry out aetiological assessments to try to discern the cause of the problem.

Identifying the cause of the hearing loss is not always possible, and in perhaps 50% of cases, it is never traced. However, every effort should be made to do this; parents can harbour a strong sense of guilt if the cause of the loss is not established. A mother and hearing impaired son recently attended one of our hearing aid review clinics. We knew the family well. The child had been deaf since birth and was now 10 years old. The mother had always appeared quite composed about the hearing loss. On this occasion, however, she suddenly burst into tears in the middle of a clinic, distraught that she had in some way caused her son's problems. For years, she had been harbouring a guilt that the deafness was all her fault. She had gradually become convinced of this because no serious attempt had been made to establish what had caused the loss, and she could do nothing else but blame it on herself.

After the initial consultations, the audiology department will need to begin regular sessions with the family, fitting hearing aids and building a clearer picture of the extent of the loss.

The family should have the opportunity to be enrolled onto a habilitation programme, often run jointly between the education and audiology services. The basic function of such a programme is to help both the child and the family to come to terms with the problem, and to help the child make maximum use of his residual hearing. The contents of such programmes are covered in later chapters.

As a final point, it is important for parents to be clear about whether other treatment could help. In these days of computers, fast communication and in particular the Internet, some parents will have done their own 'surfing' and sometimes come across very new research into hearing loss, which has not yet reached the mainstream of knowledge. Just occasionally, this has led to parents persuading the professionals to try some treatment they might not otherwise have done, with beneficial results. This is not to say that the professionals do not know what is going on but that research into hearing loss is vast and varied, and it is almost impossible for professionals to know everything on a broad front as it happens. Parents, on the other hand, will have a very sharp eye for anything that may relate to their child and can then use the professionals to put what they have found into context, to sift any real possibilities from the quackery.

Summary

To summarize this section, the following list describes features that are desirable in a comprehensive audiology service:

- a named person in charge of paediatric audiology
- specified targets for the age of identification of hearing loss
- a process for monitoring the service performance against those targets
- clearly defined procedures for screening hearing, with training and monitoring of the staff carrying out the screening (screening may include targeted or universal neonatal screening, distraction test screening, school nurse screening and vigilance)
- a clear fast-track route to assessment where there is concern
- professionals with a high level of expertise in paediatric audiology to provide assessment and follow-up programmes
- access to aetiological assessment, developmental assessment and assessment of vision
- access to genetic counselling if parents want this
- good habilitation programmes with clearly defined aims and procedures, and an approach in which the family members are equal partners in the process (and often involving professionals across a range of disciplines)
- access to whichever hearing aids are best for the child's needs
- open access for earmoulds
- hearing aid fitting programmes with clearly defined aims and goals, probably utilizing a prescription approach to fitting; if they do not, the reasons should be made clear to the parents
- ongoing monitoring of hearing aid use, with access to alternative devices if hearing aids are not successful (these may include access to radio aids, frequency transposition aids, vibrotactile aids, cochlear implants and so on)
- unbiased access, where the parents wish it, to whichever communication mode they wish to follow (signing, total communication, aural, etc.).

The key to successful habilitation is a partnership between the family and the professionals, working in a spirit of openness and backed by high-quality clinical and educational audiology facilities.

References

Baldwin M, Watkin P (1997) Diagnostic procedures. In McCracken W, Laoide-Kemp S (Eds) Audiology in Education. London: Whurr.

British Society of Audiology (1988) Recommendation: descriptors for pure-tone audiograms. British Journal of Audiology 22: 123.

Davis A, Bamford J, Wilson I, Ramkalawan T, Forshaw M, Wright S (1997) A critical review of the role of neonatal hearing screening in the detection of congenital hearing impairment. Health Technology Assessment Programme 1(10).

Ewing IR, Ewing AWG (1944) The ascertainment of deafness in infancy and early childhood. Journal of Laryngology and Otology 59: 309–38.

McCormick B (1993) Behavioural hearing tests 6 months to 5 years. In McCormick B (Ed.) Paediatric Audiology 0–5 Years, 2nd Edn. London: Whurr.

National Deaf Children's Society (1994) Quality Standards in Paediatric Audiology, Vol. I: Guidelines for the Early Identification of Hearing Impairment. London: NDCS.

National Deaf Children's Society (1996) Quality Standards in Paediatric Audiology, Vol II: The Audiological Management of the Child with Permanent Hearing Loss. London: NDCS.

Shiu J, Purvis M, Sutton G (1996) Detection of Childhood Hearing Impairment in the Oxford Region. Report of the Regional Audit Project. Oxford: Oxfordshire RHA.

Wilson WR, Thompson G (1984) Behavioural audiometry. In Jerger J (Ed.) Paediatric Audiology. London: Taylor & Francis.

Chapter 2
Causes of hearing impairment

VALERIE NEWTON AND JACQUELINE STOKES

Determining the cause of a hearing impairment is important for parents. When an unexpected disability is diagnosed in a young child, parents need an explanation – an answer to 'Why our baby? Why us?' Some parents find it hard to make progress in adapting to their hearing impaired baby's needs until a real effort has been made to find out what caused the hearing loss. Knowing the cause of the loss also becomes very important for parents when they are planning their families: they need to know the risks of having a further child with a hearing impairment. The hearing impaired child, too, will need to know, at a later date, what the risks to his own future children might be. An accurate diagnosis of the cause is also important for the community as a whole, in order that preventive measures can be introduced where available.

In this chapter, the main causes of permanent childhood hearing impairment are described and the main routes for investigating the causes outlined.

Types of hearing impairment

The first distinction to be made is between sensorineural and conductive hearing losses. Most permanent childhood hearing losses are sensorineural. This means that the damage to the hearing system lies within the cochlea, in the inner ear. The cochlea is responsible for transmitting information about incoming sound to the hearing nerve and thence to the brain. A sensorineural hearing loss affects not only a child's ability to discriminate between sounds of differing intensity, but also the ability to hear a difference between sounds of different frequency. It makes listening in noisy situations particularly difficult.

Much less frequently, the damage or defect is found in the outer ear or the middle ear, leading to a conductive hearing loss (see Chapter 1). The damage or malformation effectively makes the transfer of sound to the inner ear less efficient, causing an attenuation of sound. Conductive losses are usually in the mild-to-moderate range of hearing impairment. A conductive hearing loss mainly affects the loudness of sounds.

When the hearing loss is a result of problems in the cochlea (sensorineural loss) and in the middle and/or outer ear (conductive loss), it is described as mixed.

Hearing impairment is occasionally due to problems in the pathways that transmit signals from the cochlea to the brain, or to damage within the brain itself (i.e. retrocochlear hearing loss).

Permanent hearing loss may be present at birth (congenital) or may appear some time afterwards (acquired). This classification is not ideal because there are some congenital conditions in which the baby is born with normal hearing but develops a hearing loss during the first years of life; some inherited hearing losses are like this. They are of late onset and are progressive so that the hearing impairment may not become apparent for a number of years. The causes of hearing loss described in this chapter are organized according to whether the cause is prenatal (occurring before birth), perinatal (acquired at around the time of birth) or postnatal (acquired during childhood).

Identifying a cause

Early detection of hearing impairment followed by appropriate investigation of the causative factors gives the best chance of identifying the reasons for the hearing loss. Investigations may involve taking a detailed family history, sometimes going back several generations. Information gathered about the child's hearing impairment and the hearing of other members of the family can be extremely useful in identifying inherited hearing losses. A family history, together with a clinical examination to look for any evidence of other problems that could indicate a syndrome, is frequently the first step in determining a cause. An examination of other organs may be arranged to look for evidence of a syndrome; for example, an electro-cardiogram (ECG) will examine the function of the heart; blood and urinary examinations indicate kidney function; examination of the eyes provides evidence of abnormal pigmentation; and a scan of the inner ear shows a congenital abnormality.

Increasingly, a blood sample will be taken for DNA analysis as more genes are found that enable a definite diagnosis to be made in some genetic conditions. Referral for genetic counselling when a hereditary cause is suspected can help the family to understand the probable pattern of inheritance. This information may be of major importance to the child and his family and have implications for future family planning.

Although a large portion of childhood hearing impairment is inherited, a sizeable proportion is caused by external factors. It is important to search for external factors such as viral infections during pregnancy, for example rubella (German measles). Prematurity and low birth weight, severe jaundice, and lack of oxygen at birth are all predisposing causes. Other causes of acquired hearing loss after birth include meningitis, head injury and the use of certain medications.

Following referral for appropriate investigations, there needs to be a health professional who is responsible for conveying the results to the parents. It is important to let parents know the results of all tests and investigations, irrespective of whether they are positive or negative. Finally, that professional should draw the results together and counsel the parents on the findings at the earliest opportunity.

Unfortunately, determining the cause of a hearing impairment is not always an achievable goal. For many children with permanent hearing impairment, no cause can be found. This is for several reasons. Late diagnosis of a hearing loss may mean that even when an infective agent is found, it is not possible to be confident that it caused the hearing loss: it may simply be the result of an infection acquired during infancy. The family history may not be known in sufficient detail to allow the identification of a hereditary factor. Problems around the time of birth occur in many babies who do not develop a hearing impairment, so the presence of a traumatic birth history does not necessarily mean that this was the cause in a particular child.

Prenatal causes

Over half of all permanent childhood hearing impairments are prenatal in origin. The prenatal causes are grouped here under headings: genetic causes, congenital disorders, infections and ototoxic drugs.

Genetic causes

How is hearing loss inherited?

It is estimated that approximately 840 children are born with a permanent hearing impairment in the UK each year. About half of these hearing losses are inherited. It is important to understand the pattern in which the loss is inherited because this affects the risk of further children with hearing impairment being born into the family. Most genetic losses, about 70%, are inherited in a recessive pattern. A smaller percentage, about 25%, are inherited in a dominant pattern, the remainder being X-linked.

Recessive pattern

Figure 2.1a illustrates the recessive pattern of inheritance. The parents, who are normally hearing, each have a gene for hearing loss paired with a normal gene. A pair of genes for hearing loss is needed for the child to be hearing impaired. The baby who is hearing impaired will have inherited one gene for hearing loss from each parent, i.e. will have received a 'double dose'. With recessive inheritance, the chances of a child being hearing impaired is 1 in 4.

The risk for a normally hearing child inheriting one gene for hearing loss, like his parents, is 2 out of 3.

The risk of inheriting a hearing loss is greater when the parents are close blood relations, for example cousins. This is because they are more likely to carry the same gene for deafness than if the partner comes from outside the family.

Dominant pattern

Figure 2.1b illustrates another mode of inheritance, the dominant pattern. In this pattern, one parent has a gene for hearing impairment, paired with a normal gene. In most instances, that parent has a hearing impairment. Only one gene for hearing loss is needed for the child to be hearing impaired. The parent has a 1 in 2 chance of passing the hearing impairment on to the child irrespective of the other parent's genes.

X-linked

Figure 2.1c illustrates the X-linked pattern of inheritance. In this pattern, the mother, who is normally hearing, carries the hearing loss gene. Only boys who inherit the gene have a hearing impairment. Girls who inherit the gene become carriers but do not have a hearing impairment. The chance of the mother giving birth to a son who is hearing impaired is 1 in 2. The chance of her having a girl who will be a carrier is also 1 in 2.

These risks are a guide only, and the risks for individual families should be assessed by a geneticist.

The nature of the genetic hearing impairment

Genetic hearing loss usually affects both ears and to the same extent. It is usually present at birth, but some forms develop in childhood or later. The hearing loss is sometimes accompanied by balance problems.

With the great majority of genetic hearing impairments, no other organs are affected, i.e. the disorder is non-syndromal. Some of the genes responsible for non-syndromal hearing impairment have recently been located. This process of gene mapping is important for carrier detection and for understanding the mechanisms involved in causing hearing impairment.

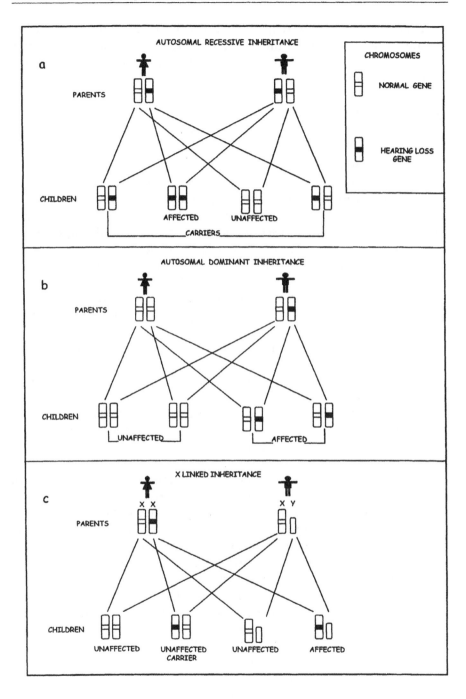

Figure 2.1 Patterns of genetic inheritance.

In a minority of children, genetic hearing impairment is accompanied by other abnormalities. In these instances, the hearing loss is part of a syndrome. It might be useful to give a brief account of some of the more familiar syndromes.

Syndromes inherited in a recessive pattern

Usher's syndrome

Usher's syndrome affects both hearing and vision. The hearing impairment is present at birth and is sensorineural. The visual impairment is caused by retinitis pigmentosa, which is a progressive condition affecting the retina at the back of the eye. The standard test of near and distant vision performed in school does not detect retinitis pigmentosa: an electroretinogram is required to make the diagnosis.

There are three types of Usher's syndrome. Together, they are believed to account for 3–6% of the congenitally deaf population.

Types 1 and 2 are by far the most common. In type 1, the hearing loss is profound, and the visual impairment appears before adolescence. In addition, there are difficulties with balance, and this is often associated with a delay in walking. Children with the type 1 syndrome may have balance problems in dim light and cling to an adult when taken out in the dark. They may also have had difficulty learning to ride a bicycle without stabilizers.

In type 2 Usher's syndrome, the hearing loss is severe and tends to be worse in the higher frequencies. The visual impairment appears after adolescence, and the balance is normal.

Type 3 syndrome is much less common. In this, the hearing loss becomes progressively worse, and balance may or may not be affected. The visual impairment appears after adolescence.

Usher's syndrome is sometimes diagnosed late, and in the meantime the child may be thought of as just rather clumsy. This is because of the way in which the eyesight is affected. Retinitis pigmentosa starts at the periphery of the eye and eventually produces tunnel vision. As a result of the deteriorating visual field, the child may stumble over objects on the floor and may have trouble tracking the ball in field games. There may also be problems with discomfort when going from darkness into a well-lit room. Eventually, it may become more apparent that these problems are due to a visual difficulty rather than clumsiness.

Six different genes are known to play a part in Usher's syndrome type 1, one of which has been located. Progress is being made towards locating and identifying all the genes for types 1, 2 and 3.

Pendred's syndrome

It is estimated that at least 4–6% of hearing impaired children have this syndrome. It is associated with a defect of the thyroid gland that leads to a goitre appearing during childhood. The hearing impairment is usually severe or profound and sensorineural in type. Some children also suffer balance problems.

A positive diagnosis is possible in some families now that a gene responsible for Pendred's syndrome has been found.

Jervell and Lange–Neilson syndrome

This is a rare syndrome that accounts for less than 1% of the population of hearing impaired children. Children with this syndrome have a profound sensorineural hearing loss and a heart defect. The heart condition may be life threatening. It is important to diagnose this condition as treatment is available using medication or a heart pacemaker. There may be episodes of altered consciousness and fainting during infancy or early childhood. Diagnosis is made by an ECG.

The gene responsible has been identified, so a positive diagnosis can be made. Parents of children with this syndrome are also advised to have ECGs as they may be prone to changes in heart rhythm.

Mucopolysaccharidoses

Hurler's syndrome, also known as MPS1, is the most common member of this group. The hearing loss is usually mixed because of substances being deposited in the middle ear. Children have learning difficulties in addition to skeletal, hearing and visual problems.

Hurler's syndrome is a progressive disorder, and there is currently no cure. A positive diagnosis can be made because the gene responsible has been found.

Syndromes inherited in a dominant pattern

Waardenburg's syndrome

This is the most common syndrome inherited in a dominant manner. Two of the genes involved have been found, which has made diagnosis of Waardenburg syndrome types 1 and 2 a possibility.

Almost all children with Waardenburg's syndrome type 1 have an unusual eye appearance and small nostrils (Figure 2.2). The eyebrows may be bushy and meet in the middle over the bridge of the nose. In both types 1 and 2, the iris of each eye may be a different colour – one blue, one brown, for example – or only a wedge-shaped portion of the iris may be a different colour. However, the most distinctive characteristic in both syndrome types is a white forelock which may be present at birth or develop in the teens. Children do not necessarily have all of the features of the syndromes even if they are in the same family.

Hearing loss is the most serious feature of this syndrome. When hearing impairment occurs, it affects one or both ears. It is sensorineural in type and may be profound in degree; one ear may be more affected than the other. The hearing loss is usually stable throughout childhood.

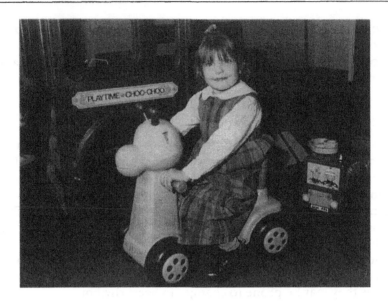

Figure 2.2 The eye appearance associated with Waardenburg's syndrome type 1.

Branchio-oto-renal syndrome

Hearing loss is the most common feature of this syndrome and may be conductive, sensorineural or mixed, but is usually mixed and severe. The hearing loss may remain stable, although in some children it deteriorates progressively.

Small pits in front of the ear and cup-shaped outer ears are the most usual outward signs. Various problems associated with the kidneys and urinary system may also be present. Children with external signs and a hearing loss should be investigated for these associated problems.

A gene responsible for this syndrome has been located, which means that the syndrome can be positively identified in some families.

Marshall Stickler syndrome

Children with this disorder have a hearing loss and various eye, skeletal and facial problems. The hearing loss is usually sensorineural, although there is sometimes a conductive component as well. Children with this condition usually have better hearing for low-frequency sounds than for sounds of higher frequency. Occasionally, the hearing gets progressively worse over the years.

Myopia (short-sightedness) is the most common eye problem, but children need close monitoring for other visual difficulties that may develop.

Some children have a cleft palate, and this is associated with a small jaw. The other mid-facial parts are sometimes also underdeveloped, which makes the face look flat.

A laxity in the joints may be found, and arthritis can develop.

Treacher Collins syndrome

As in many syndromes, the extent to which each individual is affected varies. The syndrome can be positively diagnosed as the gene responsible has been located.

Children with this syndrome may have an underdeveloped lower jaw and cheeks (Figure 2.3). Occasionally, a baby may be born with a cleft palate, which will lead to early feeding difficulties. The eyes may also be affected. They tend to slope downwards, and there is sometimes a notch along the lower edge of the eyelid.

The outer ears may be small and poorly formed. Malformation of the ear canal and middle ears may lead to a conductive type of hearing loss. These children can benefit from a hearing aid, but whether a hearing aid worn behind the ear, a body-worn aid or bone conduction aid is provided will depend on the assessment of the individual child.

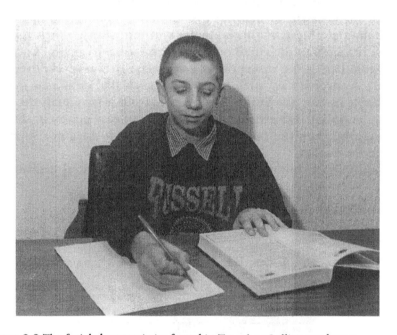

Figure 2.3 The facial characteristics found in Treacher Collins syndrome.

Syndromes inherited in X-linked pattern

Alport's syndrome

This syndrome affects both hearing and the kidneys. The kidney is affected first, the damage being progressive. The sensorineural hearing loss usually appears after 6 years of age. Hearing for the higher-frequency sounds is affected first, but the hearing loss gradually progresses. Boys are affected earlier and more severely than girls. A gene has been found for this condition.

Congenital disorders

Down's syndrome

About 1 child in 800 is born with Down's syndrome. The cause is usually an extra chromosome 21.

This is probably the most well-known congenital syndrome, and people are familiar with the distinctive characteristics of children with Down's syndrome (Figure 2.4).

Babies are often 'floppy' because of poor muscle tone, and subsequent physical development tends to be slower than normal as a result. Walking occurs relatively late. Down's syndrome children have learning difficulties and may have heart, eye and craniofacial abnormalities.

The main cause of hearing loss affecting children with Down's syndrome is 'glue ear' (otitis media with effusion), which tends to persist throughout the childhood years. The usual treatment for persistent 'glue ear' is the insertion of grommets. However, children with Down's syndrome have such narrow ear canals that grommets may not be a viable option; the fitting of two hearing aids is frequently the better treatment option. Nevertheless, this is never an easy option in children, particularly when the outer ear is so soft that it does not support a behind-the-ear aid.

About 5% of children are born with a sensorineural hearing loss,

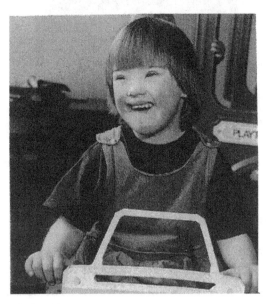

Figure 2.4 Facial features of Down's syndrome.

while a small proportion may have a conductive loss arising from the unusual development of the tiny bones in the middle ear. Some children develop a high-frequency hearing loss in their teens. It is clearly important to monitor the hearing status of these children throughout their childhood and teenage years.

Craniofacial microsomia

This is also known as first arch syndrome, hemifacial microsomia and Goldenhar's syndrome. The effects of this syndrome vary greatly, which makes accurate diagnosis difficult.

The way in which the syndrome affects the outer and middle ears is the most important factor. The outside part of the ear may be virtually absent or simply misshapen, and the external ear canal is sometimes absent (atretic). One or both ears may be affected. The middle ear, which contains the three tiny bones of hearing, may also be abnormal. As a result, sound is not conducted properly to the inner ear. Clearly, the child who has a conductive hearing loss will benefit from amplification. Judgements will have to be made on which type of hearing aid – behind-the-ear, body worn, bone conduction on a headband or bone anchored – will best meet the needs of the individual child.

Klippel–Feil anomalad

This is an uncommon condition characterized by a short neck owing to the fusion of the spine in this region. As a result, turning the head is difficult. The extent to which the spine is affected varies from child to child.

The associated hearing loss may be conductive, sensorineural or both. The outer ear may be poorly developed, the ear canal may be narrow or absent, and the middle ear may be abnormally developed, all of which leads to a significant conductive hearing loss. These children benefit from amplification, and the challenge is to fit the child with a hearing aid that fits the child's ear appropriately.

Infections

In the Western world, infections during pregnancy are nowadays much less likely to be the cause of permanent childhood hearing impairment because of immunizations and abortion for congenital rubella. Rubella infection is now an unusual cause of hearing impairment in Britain.

The TORCH test may be requested where the cause of the hearing loss is suspected to be infection during the prenatal stage. TORCH is a mnemonic for the infectious agents known to cause congenital hearing impairment, i.e. Toxoplasmosis, Rubella, Cytomegalovirus and Herpes virus.

Toxoplasmosis

This infection is not common but can lead to sensorineural hearing loss that is present at birth.

Rubella

When the infection occurs during the first weeks of pregnancy, the unborn baby is most at risk of multiple problems. Children with congenital rubella syndrome may have heart and eye defects, learning difficulties and sometimes language disorders. When the infection occurs a little later in pregnancy, the most common problem is hearing loss. This is usually sensorineural but may be mixed. The hearing loss usually affects both ears, is often severe or profound, and may become progressively worse.

Cytomegalovirus

Cytomegalovirus infection may be transmitted to the baby from the mother during pregnancy, during birth, through breast-feeding, saliva or blood transfusion, or, very unusually, through cross-infection in hospital. It is possible to test for this infection, but when the tests are carried out more than 3 weeks after birth, the chance of knowing for sure that the infection was congenital is reduced.

Hearing loss follows an infection acquired during pregnancy and is found in about 10% of children born with this infection. The loss usually affects both ears and frequently gets progressively worse. There are occasionally also learning difficulties. Some children who have had this infection appear to have entirely normal hearing on standard hearing tests yet have problems understanding what they hear.

Herpes virus

Infection with herpes virus is also known to cause sensorineural hearing loss.

Ototoxic drugs

Broadly speaking, 'ototoxic' means poisonous to the ear. There are a number of medications used that are known to have the potential to damage hearing. Streptomycin given to the mother during pregnancy may cross the placental barrier and result in a sensorineural hearing loss in the baby. Anti-malarial drugs, such as quinine, may have a similar effect on the unborn baby.

Perinatal causes

Some babies lose their hearing at or around the time of birth, about 17% of permanent hearing impairments being acquired during this perinatal period. Lack of sufficient oxygen, excessive bilirubin levels and infections can each be a cause of sensorineural hearing loss.

Babies who are premature and have a low birth weight are at greater risk of having a hearing loss than are those born at term. The number with hearing loss resulting from perinatal causes has increased as a result of better survival rates for low birth weight babies. Although the number of special care babies with a sensorineural hearing impairment is small, they tend to have additional difficulties.

When babies have breathing difficulties that require ventilation, they can be at risk of sensorineural hearing impairment. Babies who are born very prematurely, with very low birth weight, are particularly prone to problems from lack of oxygen because the immature brain is so susceptible to damage.

Many babies are born with slightly raised levels of bilirubin and are treated by phototherapy. Much less commonly, when the level of bilirubin in the blood is so high that it requires treatment by exchange transfusion, there is a risk of sensorineural hearing loss. Rhesus incompatibility is one condition associated with particularly high bilirubin levels, but this is rare nowadays as pregnant mothers at risk are given anti-D antibody.

Some babies, especially those with low birth weight, may develop infections around the time of birth. Meningitis in the first days of life may necessitate treatment with antibiotics which may damage the hearing and balance systems. The level of the antibiotic in the blood needs to be carefully monitored to avoid sustaining damage to the inner ear.

Many children who have acquired their hearing loss as a result of these perinatal causes have high-frequency hearing losses. In some children, however, the hearing loss affects all frequencies. Profound hearing loss may be found along with other major disabilities such as cerebral palsy or severe visual problems.

Postnatal causes

There are a number of ways in which hearing can be lost during childhood. Infections, particularly meningitis, are a major cause, and ototoxic drugs and trauma may also be involved.

Infections

Meningitis

Meningitis is the main cause of permanent postnatal hearing loss. It is important to recognize the chief signs of meningitis – high temperature, discomfort to light, neck stiffness and increasing drowsiness – so that treatment can be given as soon as possible.

About 10% of children with meningitis suffer a hearing loss. This is more likely following a bacterial rather than a viral infection. Several bacteria are involved in causing meningitis in children. The introduction of the HIB vaccine is expected to reduce the incidence of meningitis caused by *Haemophilus influenzae*, which is one of the most common bacteria involved. The addition of steroids to the use of antibiotics has been effective in reducing the incidence of hearing loss due to meningitis.

Hearing loss usually affects both ears. It is very occasionally progressive. There have been a few reports of improvements in hearing after meningitis, but the greater the degree of hearing loss initially, the more likely it is to persist. As children recover from the infection, many show difficulties with balance.

It is important that all children suffering from meningitis are referred for a hearing test at a paediatric audiology department. This is not only because 1 in 10 will have a hearing loss, but also because a number of these children will have such a severe hearing loss that they may benefit from a cochlear implant. Children with profound hearing losses resulting from meningitis need a rapid referral to a cochlear implant centre. This is because changes may occur in the inner ear during the healing process following meningitis that will affect the insertion of an implant (see Chapter 6).

Measles

Measles may rarely cause a moderate-to-severe sensorineural hearing loss affecting both ears. The incidence of measles has been considerably reduced in Britain as a result of vaccination. In developing countries, too, immunization programmes are helping to reduce the incidence of measles.

Mumps

Hearing loss after mumps is also now less common after the introduction of the MMR (measles, mumps and rubella) vaccination. Hearing loss as a result of mumps usually affects only one ear and is profound. Sometimes both balance and hearing are affected.

Ototoxic drugs

The potential for some drugs to damage the inner ear was mentioned above. Some powerful antibiotics, such as gentamycin, are known to be ototoxic. Children with renal disease are at risk of hearing loss as their kidneys are less efficient at removing these drugs. Their use has to be closely monitored, especially in this group of children.

Other causes of ototoxicity are the 'loop diuretics' used to control the fluid content of the body and some pharmaceutical products such as cis-platinum that are used in the treatment of childhood cancers.

Trauma

A whole variety of injuries can cause damage to the ear. A skull fracture that affects the middle ear or inner ear can cause hearing impairment. Even a minor head injury can cause a conductive hearing loss if the small bones in the middle ear are disrupted.

Summary

There are many reasons for making efforts to determine the cause of hearing impairment. For many families, it is very important to under-stand how the hearing loss has occurred in order better to cope with its effect on their lives. It also becomes important when planning further children that families are able to assess the likelihood of having another child with a hearing loss. Indeed, it becomes important for the hearing impaired child, too, when he becomes adult to understand the risks to his own children. In addition, determining the cause is of benefit to the health of the community. It is important to identify areas to target for prevention and for monitoring the effects of any measures introduced. Knowledge of the extent to which each cause is increasing or decreasing in the community helps to ensure the best use of resources, and there may be implications for the forward-planning of educational provision: some causes are associated with additional major disabilities that will require special educational provision.

This chapter has outlined some causes of permanent childhood hearing impairment. Most of these hearing losses are due to prenatal causes, and they are mainly genetic in origin. As we have seen, genetic counselling has improved in recent years as a result of research that has successfully detected causative genes. Genetic counselling should clearly be freely available to families who require it.

Unfortunately, it remains the case that the cause of many instances of childhood hearing loss goes undiscovered. Early detection of hearing impairment followed by appropriate investigation provides parents with the best chance of identifying a cause for their child's hearing impairment.

Further reading

Information on genetic conditions may be obtained from the following publications:

Gorlin RJ, Toriello HV, Cohen MM (Eds) (1995) Hereditary Hearing Loss and its Syndromes. Oxford: Oxford University Press.
Martini A, Read A, Stephens D (Eds) (1996) Genetics of Hearing Impairment. London: Whurr.

For information on current UK paediatric hearing screening practice, including the effect of early intervention on outcomes, see:

Davis A, Bamford J, Wilson I, Ramkalawan T, Wright S (1997) A critical review of the role of neonatal hearing screening in the detection of congenital hearing impairment. Health Technology Assessment 1(10).
Fortnum H, Davis A, Butler A, Stevens J (1997) Health Service Implications of Changes in Aetiology and Referral Patterns of Hearing Impaired Children in Trent 1985–1993. Report to Trent Health. Nottingham/Sheffield: MRC Institute of Hearing Research and Trent Health.

For information on risk factors for hearing loss, see:

Sutton GJ, Rowe SJ (1997) Risk factors for childhood sensorineural hearing loss in the Oxford Region. British Journal of Audiology 31: 39–54.

Family support groups

Further information on some of these causes of hearing loss and their family support networks may be obtained from:
Contact a Family
170 Tottenham Court Road
London W1P OHA
Tel: 0171–383 3555
Fax: 0171–383 0259
e-mail: info@cafamily.org.uk

Chapter 3
Audiological management in the first 18 months

ROGER GREEN

Photographs by Joanne Lazenby

Perhaps the single most important item in the habilitation of a hearing impaired child is the hearing aid. Once the diagnosis has been confirmed, and medical or surgical treatment has been ruled out, the idea of a hearing aid needs to be quickly introduced. As the age of identification gets ever younger, so the process of selecting and evaluating hearing aids becomes more and more demanding. Much of the first 18 months is spent selecting and fine-tuning hearing aids as a more and more accurate picture of the hearing loss is built up. The aim of this chapter is to throw some light on that process.

Keeping calm in the middle of an earthquake – the parent perspective

Once hearing loss is confirmed, the sooner hearing aids can be issued the better. It is important to get the child 'on the air' as soon as possible. Hearing aid issue therefore usually happens in the early days after diagnosis. Families will still be battling to come to terms with the diagnosis, and the shock and the grief that they feel may come out in a range of emotions, including sadness, anxiety, confusion and depression. They may find it impossible to accept that their child can be less than perfect and may even deny that there is a problem. Eventually, there will be recognition that the problem is real, but this may come very gradually. Emotions may turn to guilt or anger. Parents may find themselves looking for someone to blame: themselves, the doctors, the nurses, the audiology team, even the phases of the moon. They may have a sense of helplessness and isolation. They will look for any sign from the professionals that things are not as bad as first thought. A tiny improvement in one test result may send them away from a test session elated with relief

55

and hope, hope that can easily turn to despair when the improvement is not maintained.

Most parents finally come to accept their child's disability. The feeling of crisis fades, and the healing starts. They come to recognize that their child is different, but only because he cannot hear. Because of the hearing loss, he will have to work harder in the area of language. Otherwise, he has just the same appetite for life as any other child:

> Ken is deaf but he is normal in every other way – he plays with the dog, is happy to see me and Dad, and is a crazy kind of kid. (Adams, 1991)

Even when acceptance gradually emerges, parents will find themselves cycling back through the whole range of emotions, taking two steps forward and one back.

Against this stormy background, the clinician is trying to fit hearing aids, explaining their use and care, and expecting the parents quickly to become experts in hearing aid management. The clinician understands the need for the aid and the benefits that it will bring. The parents may hate it. It is the first visible proof that their child has a real problem, that the experts have not got it wrong, that this is something permanent. It is a monstrous chunk of plastic, hung from their child's ear and advertising to the whole world that their child is disabled. It is not surprising that some parents find it very difficult to accept the hearing aid calmly at first. They don't like to look at it, to touch it, even to have it in the house. Little surprise then that the early months of hearing aid use may not be a smooth passage.

The clinician needs to proceed with hearing aids as soon as is reasonably possible. He must, however, continue to be extremely alert and sensitive to the feelings of the parents. While the parents need to understand the importance of the hearing aids, they should still lead the process. Indeed, if they are still too much in shock and not yet ready to cope with hearing aids, it may be better to delay fitting them and concentrate on supporting the parents until they feel ready to proceed.

'What good is a hearing aid if my child can't hear?' – what hearing aids do

Very few children are totally deaf. If a child really cannot hear anything at all, it is true that a hearing aid will provide no benefit – except possibly a sense of touch as the child feels the vibration in his ear. Most children can hear something; it is just that the sound must be very intense before the ear will detect it. The purpose of a hearing aid is to amplify sound so that it reaches the ear at a level that the ear can detect. (In the same way, some children with partial vision can only see bright lights. Vision aids can take normal light and make it bright enough for the eye to detect.) A hearing aid is an extraordinary device. With it, children, even those who have very severe hearing losses, can learn to make sense of the world of sound and turn what they hear into speech.

This feat is even more remarkable when one considers the nature of cochlear hearing loss. When the cochlea is damaged, the hearing is affected in a number of ways. We have already discussed the fact that it only responds to louder sounds. Another problem is that of distortion. Even sounds that can be heard will sound different from what a normal hearing person experiences. One way to think of this is to imagine playing a tape on a tape recorder with dirty playback heads, or a record on a record player with a needle covered in fluff. The sound you hear is probably quiet, muffled and distorted. Wearing a hearing aid is equivalent to increasing the volume. The sound will be louder but still muffled and distorted.

Despite this, a child can learn to turn that muffled and distorted sound into words. The secret is to get the aid correctly tuned as early as possible and to encourage the child to wear the aid as much as possible. Consistent and continuous aid use is a powerful ally in the development of speech and language.

How long should we wait before trying hearing aids?

Once a loss is confirmed, hearing aids should be fitted as soon as possible. The National Deaf Children's Society (NDCS) Quality Standards (1994) suggest that they be issued within 4 weeks. There are some qualifications to this, however. As has already been said, some parents are reluctant to accept hearing aids. It may be appropriate to delay fitting hearing aids for a short time in order to give the family more time to come to terms with the hearing loss and the fact that it is a long-term problem. With milder losses, the effects of the loss will not be as noticeable, and parents may need a lot of convincing that there really is a problem. With such losses, hearing aid issue is still important but its timing not quite as critical, so a short delay before fitting is perhaps more common in this situation. Where severe or profound deafness is suspected, every effort should be made to help the family come to terms with hearing aids and thus enable early fitting to take place. However, the problem is often more obvious with this degree of loss, so parents are more prepared to act quickly.

'How do you know which aid to fit?' – hearing aid selection

Hearing aids are mainly designed to help a child detect speech. We therefore want a hearing aid that amplifies most where the speech frequencies are poorest. But how much amplification is optimum? It sounds like a simple question, but much has been written on the subject (e.g. Byrne, 1983; Byrne and Dillon, 1986; Seewald, 1992) without a completely clear answer emerging. The obvious answer turns out to be the wrong answer. If a child has a loss of 70 dB at 1000 Hz, you might think that the best solution is to set the aid to amplify 1000 Hz by 70 dB.

There are various problems with this idea. One is a problem known as recruitment, which often accompanies cochlear damage. The ear is a very sophisticated organ; it can do many clever things. When it works well, it can detect very quiet sounds. It can also put up with very loud sounds. However, the process that detects quiet sounds is not the same as the process that controls loud sounds. When the cochlea is damaged, it may not process quiet sounds, but it may still respond strongly to loud sounds. If a hearing aid amplifies sounds to a level that is too loud, the child will experience frequent discomfort and may reject the aid.

Even if tolerating loud sounds is not a problem, other factors prevent us from simply making hearing aids more and more powerful. There are physical limits on how much a hearing aid can amplify and levels beyond which too much vibration of the ear would become hazardous. Because of this, there is a power ceiling beyond which hearing aids cannot go.

So, we need to fit a hearing aid that makes speech sounds audible but does not give the child discomfort. How do we go about this?

Figure 3.1 shows an audiogram chart on which are shown the average levels of typical speech sounds at different frequencies, spoken at a distance of 2 metres – note that speech tends to be naturally louder in the

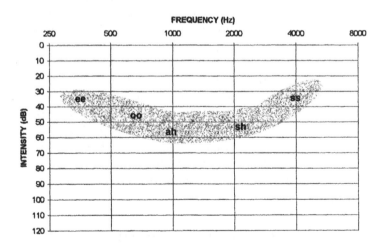

Figure 3.1 Audiogram showing levels and frequencies of selected speech sounds. Note that the intensity of speech is constantly varying across the range of levels represented by the shaded area.

low frequencies than in the high frequencies. Thus the vowel sound 'a' contains frequencies of around 1000 Hz and in normal conversation is typically about 60 dB loud. The consonant sound 'ss' is higher in frequency, containing frequencies of around 4000 Hz. It is also a lot less intense in normal speech, with typical levels of about 40 dB. Of course, these sound levels vary during the course of a conversation. (This is a very simplified account, and a fuller description can be found in Ling, 1989.)

Figure 3.2 shows an audiogram for a child with a moderate hearing loss. Essentially, we want to fit a hearing aid that improves the hearing thresholds to a level at which the speech sounds can be heard. At the same time, we do not want to raise the levels so much that the child finds louder sounds uncomfortable.

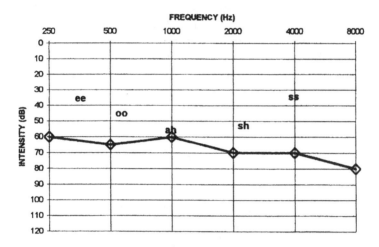

Figure 3.2 Audiogram from a child with moderate hearing loss.

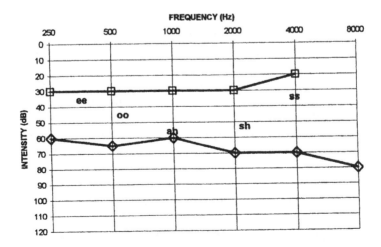

Figure 3.3 Audiogram from a child with moderate hearing loss, also showing the aided thresholds. ◇ = free-field thresholds unaided; □ = free-field thresholds aided.

In Figure 3.3 on page 59, a set of aided thresholds is also shown. If we can fit a hearing aid that lets the child hear this well, he should be able to hear all the sounds of speech. We can calculate the amount of amplification at each frequency by subtracting the unaided thresholds from the required aided thresholds. The result is shown below:

FREQUENCY	250 Hz	500 Hz	1000 Hz	2000 Hz	4000 Hz
AMPLIFICATION	30 dB	35 dB	30 dB	40 dB	50 dB

The clinician can then select and tune a hearing aid to give that degree of amplification.

Parents often ask, 'Why not just wind up the hearing aid so that all the thresholds are at 0 dB – he could then hear like a normal hearing child?' The simple answer to this question is the one given above. For some children, this would be too much amplification, and many sounds would be uncomfortable. We are trying to put all the sounds of speech into the child's 'comfort zone', which is usually between their threshold and about 110 dB.

There is also a more complex answer. Much research has gone into selecting the best hearing aid amplification for a given hearing loss. The amount of amplification depends on a number of factors, such as how you interpret the idea of comfort zone, which speech spectrum you use (should you use male or female? – the female spectrum is higher frequency; should you use a lower level spectrum for infants? – they spend much of their time relatively close to Mum or Dad, so the speech is already louder to them) and so on.

Some hearing aid philosophies have looked at the factors in detail and developed 'prescriptions' for what a hearing aid should do based on the audiogram. There are many of these, but two in particular have been well researched and are in more common usage. One is the prescription of the National Acoustical Laboratories in Australia (Byrne and Dillon, 1986). This has been developed from what is known about hearing-impaired psychoacoustics, although much of the research is based on adults and older children. The other is the Dynamic Sensation Level (DSL) approach of Seewald (1992), developed in the USA. This is based on children rather than adults and is becoming increasingly used in the UK. Whatever prescription approach is used, allowance needs to be made for the different requirements of conductive and sensorineural hearing losses. In brief, this means that a conductive hearing loss needs more power than the equivalent sensorineural loss because the sound from the hearing aid must 'blast its way through the blockage' to reach the inner ear.

It is clear how all this can quickly become an impenetrable maze for the parents, which is partly why we have clinicians, of course. Some parents will want to know in great detail what is going on; others will be happy to let the clinicians sort out the tricky stuff as long as they have an overview of what is happening. The NDCS Quality Standards (1996) suggested that audiology departments should be specific about the aims of the hearing aid fitting procedure, and this should at some stage be discussed with the parents.

'How do you know what to fit when you don't know how well he can hear?' – matching hearing aids to hearing tests

This is a good question. Information about the degree of hearing loss is usually limited until the child is at least 6 months old. Therefore, in the early stages, we have to make an educated guess. The whole process of hearing aid review, which means reassessing the child repeatedly once the aid is fitted, is a process of moving from guesswork to certainty as a complete picture of the hearing loss gradually evolves.

The choice of initial aid is based on at least some information. When the hearing loss is confirmed, this will be on the basis of one or more (preferably more!) test results, which give some idea of the hearing levels. Sometimes the only early results are an auditory brainstem response (ABR) threshold and some information on behavioural observation audiometry (BOA). If a child shows no response to ABR and no sign of any reaction to loud sounds, an aid would be selected which had moderate power and more or less equal amplification for all frequencies. Note, however, that it is often a good idea to give some extra boost to the high frequencies whatever the hearing loss, and most hearing aids do this.

It is wise to err on the side of caution and not fit too powerful an aid at this stage. Too much volume can distress the child and cause the aid to be rejected. Powerful hearing aids also 'whistle' in the ear more easily, so can be difficult to manage. However, too little volume is also a problem. If the aid is not powerful enough, the child will not hear with it. In terms of his experience, he now has a piece of plastic in his ear where he did not have one before. He gets nothing from this piece of plastic, so he rejects it. In order to make sure that the aid is at least broadly right, giving neither too little and nor too much amplification, it is necessary to check it frequently in the early weeks, particularly with babies.

If a child shows thresholds around 80 dB for ABR and clear waking responses to low-frequency sounds, the clinician will assume a loss that is greater in the high-frequency range. He will then fit an aid that gives more high-frequency emphasis.

As the clinician gets to know the child better, and gets more information about the hearing loss, the aid can be constantly fine-tuned or even changed altogether. The NDCS Quality Standards (1996) suggest that frequency-specific thresholds should be obtained by 1 year of age and ear-specific thresholds by 18 months. Insert earphones, which were discussed in Chapter 1, are becoming important tools in helping to achieve these ear-specific measurements early. By 30 months of age, many children will accept headphones and, through play audiometry, give clear and precise measures of hearing threshold.

How do hearing aids work?

There is a wide range of hearing aids differing in size, colour, shape, where they are worn, how much power they have and how they process sound. However, all hearing aids have certain features in common, which will be described in this section (see Figure 3.4).

Microphone

A hearing aid has a small microphone whose job is to catch the sound and convert it into electricity.

Amplifier

The hearing aid casing houses the amplifier. This amplifier collects the sound from the microphone and makes it louder. Amplifiers can also filter the sound so that some frequencies are amplified more than others. Amplifiers can be more or less powerful. Some have ways of controlling loud sound, preventing it from becoming louder than a preset level. Some amplifiers (in particular, digital amplifiers) can carry out very sophisticated processing of the sound. The clinician can tune the amplifier to match the specific needs of each individual child. This is done by making adjustments either to controls on the hearing aid itself or through a small programming box.

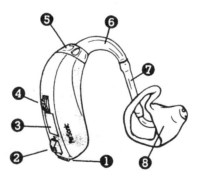

Figure 3.4 Diagram of a hearing aid. 1 = battery drawer; 2 = on–off switch; 3 = panel covering tuning controls (adjusted by the clinician); 4 = volume control; 5 = microphone; 6 = earhook; 7 = earmould tubing; 8 = earmould.

Receiver

This is like a small loudspeaker that receives the amplified and processed sound from the amplifier and directs it towards the ear.

Earhook

This is a small hook, screwed on to the hearing aid, to which the earmould attaches. Most hearing aids come with a range of earhooks, each giving a slightly different frequency response.

Earmould

This has several functions. It takes the sound from the receiver and feeds it, through a tube, down into the ear canal. It also helps to keep the aid in place at the ear. In conjunction with the earhook and earmould tubing, it can further change the sound from the hearing aid to match the needs of the child.

Battery

All hearing aids are battery operated. Batteries come in various shapes and sizes, and are nearly always of the zinc–air type. Mercury batteries should not normally be used in hearing aids as they are more dangerous if swallowed. Battery locking compartments should always be fitted to hearing aids so that young children cannot get at the battery and swallow it. Some hearing aids work only on rechargeable batteries.

On–Off switch

Most hearing aids have a switch that enables the user to turn them on and off. This switch may have other facilities such as a tone control or telecoil.

Volume control

Most hearing aids have a volume control so that the user can make the sound louder or softer. The ideal setting for this needs to be carefully chosen. Volume control covers can usually be given to avoid little fingers tampering with the control.

Feedback

This is an unwanted problem with hearing aids. In my own misspent youth in a band, much time was spent avoiding feedback, the loud howling noise that comes when the sound from the loudspeakers gets back into the guitar amplifier, or indeed, as musical fashions changed, using it for dramatic effect. Hearing aid feedback is the same. Whenever sound from the receiver leaks back into the hearing aid, feedback can occur, causing the aid to whistle. The most common cause of feedback is a poorly fitting earmould or an earmould that has been wrongly inserted or become dislodged (the sound can then leak out from inside the ear canal and get back into the hearing aid).

'I want one of those invisible ones!'

Hearing aids vary widely. Two hearing aids can look very similar but actually do very different things. Alternatively, two hearing aids can look very different but actually do nearly the same. Furthermore, each hearing aid is individually tuned to suit a particular child. Because of this, hearing aids are not interchangeable. (That is not to say that they do not get interchanged – children sometimes seem inquisitive to try each other's aids. Children even come to the clinic wearing their best friend's hearing aid, a practice definitely to be discouraged!)

This section will describe the different types of aid and then discuss which aids may best suit which children.

Behind-the-ear hearing aids

Behind-the-ear (BTE) hearing aids (or postaurals as they are sometimes known) are the most common form of hearing aid issued to children in the UK. Figures 3.5 and 3.6 show typical examples. BTEs can be anything from very low power to very high power. The aid rests behind the ear. The sound from the receiver is fed down through the earhook, which is connected to a flexible tube on the child's earmould so that the sound can be fed down to the ear canal.

When an earmould or hearing aid is changed, or when a hearing aid is returned from being repaired, it is important to make sure that the correct volume control, hearing aid settings, earhook and earmould tubing are used.

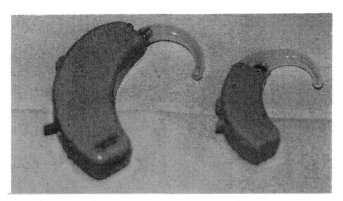

Figure 3.5 A large (high-powered) and a small (medium-powered) behind-the-ear hearing aid.

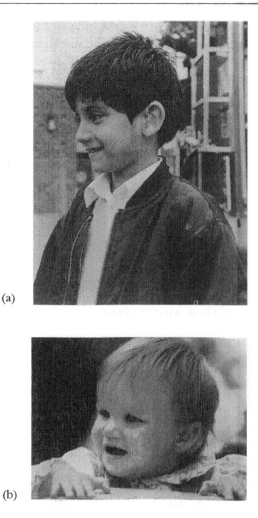

(a)

(b)

Figure 3.6 Children wearing behind-the-ear hearing aids.

Body-worn hearing aids

Figures 3.7 and 3.8 show examples of body-worn hearing aids. The microphone and amplifier are contained in a box (similar to a personal stereo) that is worn on the body. The sound is then fed by leads to a receiver that is directly connected to the earmould.

Most parents are not keen on body-worn systems as they are more cumbersome and more visible. Their main advantage over BTEs is that they can be made a little more powerful. They are also useful for very young babies, who spend much of their time in a cot. In this situation, a BTE is easily dislodged, and the hearing aid tends to whistle very easily. If the baby is wearing a body-worn hearing aid, the aid can be moved well away from the ear, perhaps clipped to the side of the cot, so that feedback is less of a problem. However, there are disadvantages to this arrangement. In particular, the child will not hear his own voice as clearly if it is a long way from the microphone.

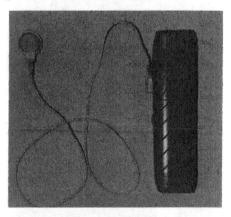

Figure 3.7 An example of a body-worn hearing aid.

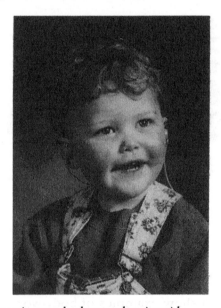

Figure 3.8 A child wearing two body-worn hearing aids.

In-the-ear hearing aids

In an in-the-ear (ITE) aid, the amplifier is built into the earmould so that the whole hearing aid sits in the ear. This obviously has much cosmetic appeal because the aid is less visible. It also has the advantage that there is only one piece of plastic, which is therefore easier to get in and out.

There are, however, some serious disadvantages with ITEs, so much so that they are seldom the right choice for very young children. First, they cannot be made very powerful – there is not enough space in the mould for all the electronics, and even if there were, feedback would be a huge problem. They are therefore only suitable for mild losses. Second, because feedback is such a problem, it is important to keep the 'mould' a good, tight fit. For infants, who grow very rapidly, new moulds need to be made even weekly, and for ITEs this can mean sending the whole hearing aid away to be rebuilt. This is both prohibitively expensive and means that the child will often be without the aid. Children with milder losses may well be able to move on to ITEs as they get older and the ear has stopped growing. It is even quite useful to hold this plan in reserve, in anticipation of their becoming self-conscious teenagers and suddenly very reluctant to wear hearing aids at all.

One version of the ITE is the in-the-canal aid, where the whole hearing aid is built into a mould that is fitted deep into the canal. These have all the problems of ITEs only more so.

Bone conduction hearing aids

For children with conductive hearing loss, the loss is caused by a blockage preventing the sound from reaching the cochlea. An example of this is canal atresia, in which the outer ear has not formed properly and part of the ear canal is replaced by solid bone or cartilage. In this case, a bone conduction hearing aid may be the most useful aid to fit. An example is shown in Figure 3.9.

The amplifier can be either a body-worn or a behind-the-ear system. Instead of the normal receiver, the patient wears a bone conductor. This rests against the head, usually behind the ear, and transfers the sound through the skull to the cochlea by direct vibration. The unit can be kept in place by a metal band across the head or, as shown in Figure 3.9, be attached to a soft, elastic headband.

A recent innovation in bone conduction hearing aids is the bone-anchored hearing aid. In order to get a good connection between the bone conductor and the skull, it is possible to implant a small screw into the thick bone of the skull and fit the bone conductor into this. A special bone conductor is used, which also houses the amplifier and microphone. It is cosmetically appealing because it is small and can be hidden behind the hair. Bone-anchored hearing aids are not suitable for very young children as the skull is not sufficiently hardened to take the fitting.

Bone-conduction hearing aids tend to be fitted when the conductive part of the loss is large (as in canal atresia) or when the ear has persistent discharge, which could be aggravated by an earmould. Milder conductive losses usually do well with ordinary hearing aids.

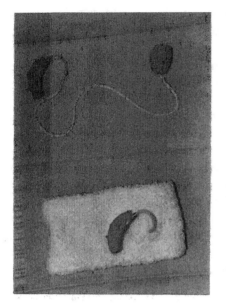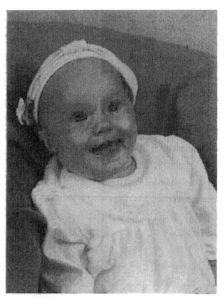

Figure 3.9 An example of a bone-conductor aid attached to an elastic headband. The top left of the picture shows a hearing aid connected to the bone vibrator. At the bottom left is the hearing aid attached to the outside of the headband by Velcro. The bone vibrator is attached to the inside, also by Velcro. The picture on the right shows a child wearing the aid.

Cochlear implants

There will be some children for whom a hearing aid is not the answer. If children have very severe hearing loss, and have tried hard with hearing aids but are still not getting enough sound, it may be appropriate to consider a cochlear implant.

Cochlear implants have been given the image of 'bionic ears', and it is tempting to think of them as miracle cures for deafness. In reality, this is far from the case. Generally, children who are successful hearing aid wearers do better to stay with their hearing aids, and cochlear implants are considered only after every effort has been made with hearing aids. There is still a good deal of debate about cochlear implants and which patients are likely to benefit from them (see, for example, Archbold, 1997, National Deaf Children's Society, 1992).

Radio hearing aids

With radio aids (also known as FM systems because they operate using frequency-modulated radio signals), the mother wears a special trans-mitter microphone. This microphone is close to her mouth so picks up mostly the sound of her voice. The child wears a radio receiver. This receiver picks up sound directly from the transmitter microphone. The transmitter and receiver communicate by a radio link, so that there are no wires connecting the two (it is rather like a high-quality walkie-talkie system). The sound from the receiver is fed to the child either through the child's hearing aid or through a small earphone connected to the earmould. Figures 3.10, 3.11 and 3.12 show examples of radio aids.

Radio hearing aids have been developed to get around one of the main problems experienced by the hearing impaired – the problem of background noise. A child sits in the kitchen while his mother prepares the dinner. She talks to the child continuously, telling the child what she is doing, perhaps letting him help. The hearing aid is picking up not only the mother's voice, but also all the background noises: saucepans, spoons, mixing bowls, the clatter of cutlery. It is difficult for the aid to separate the speech from the noise, and the child may struggle to hear.

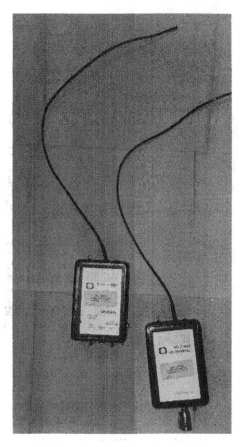

Figure 3.10 An example of a radio aid (FM) system. The parent or teacher wears one half (the transmitter) and the child the other half (the receiver). Sound from the receiver is usually fed to the child's hearing aids by a lead that plugs into the aids. See also Figures 3.11 and 3.12.

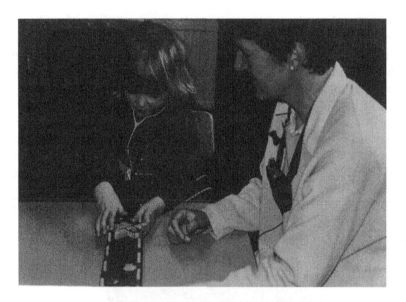

Figure 3.11 A child wearing a radio aid. Here, the teacher's transmitter and the child's receiver (packed into a soft case), and the leads to the hearing aids, can be seen.

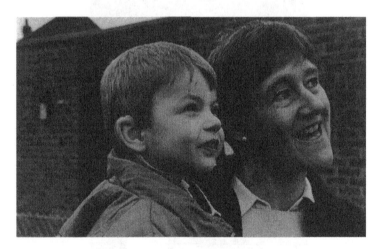

Figure 3.12 A child wearing a radio aid. The child's leads can be seen plugged into the hearing aids.

When a radio aid is used, the transmitter is mainly picking up just the mother's voice, so that this is all that the child hears: the troublesome background noise is not detected. This gives the child a better chance of hearing his mother's voice more clearly.

Radio aids have both advantages and disadvantages. They are usually used in combination with the child's hearing aid, and careful consideration is needed before the decision is made to try one.

'...Yes, but he loves custard'

So far, we have discussed only the technical aspects of hearing aids, in particular their acoustic (sound-processing) properties. It must not be forgotten that hearing aids are worn on little ears, and little ears are fixed to little heads and bodies, and the owners of those little heads and bodies like to experiment with sand or water or jam, and to see how messy stewed prunes can really be, and to practise the art of hanging upside down from climbing frames, and to see if dogs like hearing aids...

Hearing aids lead the life of Riley (see Figure 3.13). Keeping them on can be particularly tricky with children. Having a well-fitting earmould and making sure that a BTE fits snugly behind the ear can help. Other tricks can be tried. 'Huggies' are plastic loops that fit round the ear and to which the aids can be fitted. Double-sided sticky tabs can be used that stick to the aid and to the skin, keeping the aid firmly in place. Some clinics use toupee tape for the same purpose.

Body-worn hearing aids are particularly prone to filling up with breakfast, or vomit, or water, because they are worn on the child's body. Protection for the microphone can be achieved with a cover that usually fits over the microphone (without blocking it) and the volume control and switches.

To avoid children tampering with the volume control on a BTE, a cover can be fitted which only the parent can remove.

An essential for infants is a battery drawer lock. This prevents the child from opening the battery drawer and getting at the battery. Hearing aids now almost always use zinc–air batteries rather than the more

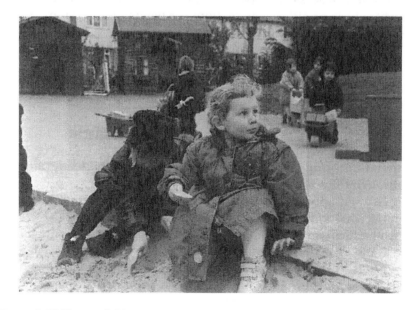

Figure 3.13 The sandpit!

poisonous mercury battery. If a battery is swallowed, it can still burn the stomach and may need surgical removal.

Finally the decor. Children delight in decorating hearing aids, and brightly coloured hearing aids are becoming very popular. The current trend is for translucent colours that allow the workings of the hearing aid to be seen through the case, and for coloured see-through watches. It is even possible to have matching hearing aids and earmoulds. Green see-through hearing aids and matching green glitter earmoulds made a much-loved combination for one child on our list. Another child wears two BTEs with a yellow side and a blue side. That way, he can swap the aids between ears to reveal yellow or blue hearing aids to match his clothes. Younger children also like to put coloured stickers all over their hearing aids. Some hearing aid companies supply sets of these (with illustrations of everything from sea horses to sunglasses). There are even examples of hearing aids designed or decorated to act as fashion items, just as spectacles can be.

Some parents are happy with bright colours. Others would rather use the colour to camouflage the aid as much as possible. It is worth noting in this regard that hearing aids are better camouflaged if their colour matches the hair colour rather than the skin colour. Hearing aids are available in blacks, greys, browns and beiges to suit these needs.

Pulling it all together

It is clear from what has been said that fitting a hearing aid is a complex and gradual process. The process takes place around what are often known as hearing aid review sessions, or habilitation sessions. So what can be expected from these sessions?

There are various interacting strands to the habilitation process:

- the ongoing assessment of the child's unaided hearing
- the prescription, selection and evaluation of the hearing aids
- the monitoring of the child's middle ear status
- the assessment of the child's use of his aided hearing
- the assessment of the child's communication skills
- the monitoring of the rate and quality of the child's development through the stages of language
- reviews at appropriate times of their mode of communication (e.g. aural, total communication or signing)
- at all stages working with parents and families to develop their expertise and enable them to take the lead role in their child's welfare
- supporting parents through difficult periods
- deciding on alternative strategies when appropriate (e.g. referral for cochlear implant assessment).

Habilitation sessions need input from professionals with a range of skills, in both hearing assessment/hearing aid issues and early language development. There will need to be input when necessary from ENT staff, paediatricians, geneticists and, where children have other learning difficulties, staff with skills in relevant specialist areas. Where English is not the first language, or not spoken with reasonable fluency, it may be necessary to arrange for interpreters to be included in the sessions. It is essential that good links exist between these clinicians. If not, the parents will find themselves acting as go-betweens. This should not happen. The parents have enough to do worrying about their child; they should not have to worry about the clinicians as well.

The remainder of this chapter will deal principally with the hearing aid review aspect of the habilitation process. Other aspects will be picked up in different chapters.

'What happens at hearing aid review?'

The first hearing aid review may be the first opportunity to sit down and discuss at length what is known about the child. All the test results, and reports from other professionals, can be pulled together and discussed with the parents. Also, a long-term plan for the child will be discussed and agreed. Typically, this will involve the parents being clear about the need for, and happy to accept, the trial of hearing aids. The process of selecting and fitting the aids, and the need for repeat visits (usually frequent at first, possibly with weekly contact, but becoming less frequent as information becomes more comprehensive and accurate) is explained. It is useful, where possible, to provide written information to give the parents to take away and browse through in their own time at home.

It is necessary to cultivate an atmosphere of openness and honesty, and to allow the parents to ask questions, even awkward questions, without fear of being thought difficult or stupid. There are many corners of audiology where unanswered questions lurk, and even the professionals do not know it all. The parent is much more likely to trust a clinician who honestly says, 'I don't know' than one who hides his ignorance behind a smoke-screen of technical jargon.

At an early stage, the first ear impressions need to be taken so that earmoulds can be manufactured. Earmoulds and their manufacture form a wide topic (Brett and Joshua, 1997). The impression must be made using correct techniques and materials. There is a range of materials available (condensation silicones, addition silicones, instant cure etc.), each of which is useful in different situations. Parents are told which materials are being used and why. The same is true of the earmould: there is a wide variety of types (open, skeleton, shell, etc.), materials (acrylic, silicone, coe, etc.) and plumbing procedures (venting, damping, high-frequency horns, etc.), all of which need to be selected on the basis of the needs of the individual child. Again, the choice of mould is explained to the parents, as is the need for sufficiently frequent impression-taking to maintain a good fit and thus control of feedback.

Before the hearing aid is fitted, the clinician will need to decide which hearing aid and hearing aid settings to start with. First, he must prescribe the amplification characteristics he thinks are right. This may not be a very precise prescription at this stage as the information from the test results is not very precise. Hearing aid prescriptions have been described above, and the particular prescription used will depend on which philosophy the clinician follows.

Having chosen the prescription, the clinician must then decide on the best aid to start with and also the aid accessories. All children under 18 months of age must have battery locks fitted if the aid is a BTE. They should also have volume control covers. The clinician may choose to fit a body-worn aid on a very young baby if difficult management problems are anticipated with a BTE.

Having selected the aid, he will set it using the internal settings on the aid so that the aid gives the amplification characteristics required. These include both the amount of gain and the maximum levels to which loud sound is allowed to rise. The clinician will check the amount of amplification by running the aid through a test box, a special box with a sound-proof chamber. The aid is placed inside it, connected to a small, artificial 'ear' (called a coupler). Different sounds are played into the hearing aid, and the amount of amplification (or gain) produced by the hearing aid is measured, as well as the maximum volume. A test box printout is shown in Figure 3.14. If the aid does not quite match the prescription, it can be reset and rechecked in the test box until a better match is achieved.

When the earmoulds are ready and the aid has been selected and set up, the child can be fitted. This can be a traumatic session and needs to be handled with great sensitivity. The parents are now face to face with the reality of their child's deafness. It can be a difficult fact to bear, and, despite outward appearances, they may take in little of what is said to them. The fitting session should concentrate on the fitting alone and not be a session in which testing is also attempted. There is far too much to do in familiarizing the parents with the aid, with explaining its workings and with getting them to practise insertion several times until they are confident. Explanation is given about the length of time the aid should be worn and about ways of gradually building up this wear time.

It is a good idea to issue a hearing aid 'passport', a booklet that covers all the settings and accessories that accompany the aid. This allows for updating as settings, and even hearing aids, change. It should clearly show the position of the settings that the parent controls, particularly the volume control, as this alone will have a significant effect on what the child hears.

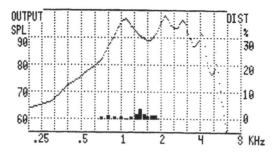

Figure 3.14 A printout of the response of a hearing aid measured in a test box. In this printout, the hearing aid is set at the volume control setting used by the child. The sound fed into the hearing aid is at 60 dB. The sound produced by the hearing aid varies with frequency, and the response is quite 'wavy', which is typical of many hearing aids. The small black columns represent the amount of distortion that the hearing aid produces. This should always be well below 10%.

When the aid goes home with the child for the first time, it is a good idea to arrange for someone to visit the family at home within a few days to make sure that all is going well. In many districts, the health and education services work closely together: the audiologist informs the education team that aids have been issued, and someone from the team arranges to visit.

It is useful for the parents to observe their child's responses to sound with and without the aid at home. Indeed, it may be worth keeping a formal diary recording any responses, for example:

- Does the child startle to loud noises?
- Does the child use his own voice more when wearing the hearing aid?
- Can you get the child's attention more easily when he is wearing his hearing aid?
- Does he hear music/the telephone/the doorbell/the vacuum cleaner/the dog barking...?
- What kind of responses does your child make to sound – smile/still/turn/dance/laugh/cry...?

However, this advice comes with two important cautions. First, observe but do not keep testing the child's responses: it is better if testing is left to the clinic. Second, don't be despondent if the aid does not produce immediate and dramatic changes. Hearing aids very seldom do. Normal-hearing children take almost a year to start making sense of the sounds that they hear. It is important to realize that hearing impaired children need time as well. Parents do not always appreciate this at first and can quickly become discouraged, losing any enthusiasm they may have had for hearing aids.

At the next hearing aid review, the clinician discusses with parents their progress with the hearing aids, their thoughts/concerns/worries/

fears about the aids and any positive results of the child being aided (even if only the fact that he kept them in for half an hour before throwing them at the dog). The clinician needs to be realistic but positive in his encouragement. Early progress can be hard to come by, and even apparently small steps may in fact be massive ones. The family is usually supported at home by a visiting teacher of the deaf, who plays a vital role in helping the parents to judge progress in the real world beyond the clinic. The teacher of the deaf gets to know the family well and uses his experience of hearing impaired children to support the parents throughout the early months of hearing aid use.

Comments about aided responses at home can be very useful in deciding whether the aid is correctly set. For example, if there has been no response at all to sound, the aid's power may need to be increased, albeit conservatively at this early stage. If the child has become jumpy and distressed with the aid, the amplification may be too loud or the maximum output set too high.

The clinician checks the aids through the test box to make sure that they are working well, always using fresh batteries for this and any subsequent testing. The ears are inspected with an otoscope. The state of the ear canal and drum is examined. If excessive wax is present in the canal, it may need to be removed. This can be a source of immense frustration for the parents, who may assume that the clinician can remove it himself. Unfortunately, wax removal is a potentially hazardous process if not carried out by someone trained in the skills. Audiologists (even very eminent ones) are not usually trained in wax removal, and the child may therefore need a trip to the ENT consultant for this. A good alternative is to have a nurse on the team trained in dewaxing techniques. It may then be possible to remove the wax straight away.

Impedance testing is carried out to check the status of the middle ears. Note that impedance testing can sometimes be misleading with very young babies, so the results must be interpreted with caution. One episode of flat impedance traces (suggesting middle ear fluid) is not a disaster, but if the condition persists, a trip to the ENT consultant may again be necessary.

For children with severe or profound losses, the effect of a temporary conductive loss because of middle ear fluid may be more serious. They may go from hearing something to effectively hearing nothing. If they are already relying on powerful hearing aids at high volume settings, they will not be able to compensate by turning up the volume still further. These children may need to be seen by ENT personnel as a priority if the condition does not quickly resolve.

If all else is well, the clinician may decide to test the child with the hearing aids on. Many of the procedures described in Chapter 1 can be used. The method used will depend on the child's age, his developmental ability and the information required. In the early stages, and with very young children, testing can be a frustrating exercise. Responses can be difficult to elicit (not least because the child is still not used to sound). In these early stages, all that can sometimes be achieved is to make sure that the aid is not giving too much gain, by checking that the child is not upset by loud sounds.

Some clinics also like to carry out what are called 'real-ear' measurements on the child once he is wearing hearing aids. This is done by putting a narrow, flexible tube into the ear. The tube is connected to a 'probe' microphone that can measure the sound levels in the ear canal itself. Probe tube measurements can be made with and without the hearing aid on in order to get a measure of what amplification the hearing aid is producing in the child's own ear. The argument for doing this is that all ears are different. When a hearing aid is measured in a test box, the aid is attached to a small cylinder, or 'coupler', which behaves like an average ear. Individual ears will all be slightly different from the coupler, so the hearing aid will respond differently as well. Also, a coupler is designed around the average adult ear. The smaller ears of babies tend to give different responses, particularly at high frequencies, at which they give more gain than the coupler would predict (Green, 1993). Real-ear measurements enable the clinician to look at the response of the hearing aid and earmould when worn on the child's ear.

Another kind of real-ear measurement can be used in the DSL prescription fitting procedure mentioned above. In this method, probe tube microphones are used along with insert earphones to measure the difference between the coupler response and the response of the child's ear. This 'real ear to coupler difference' is then used to correct any subsequent coupler measurements (Seewald, 1992).

While these real-ear measurements can be useful, the most important measurements are those which show how well the child is hearing. Until we know that, we have no reference from which to select hearing aids in the first place or to check that the child is really experiencing what we want him to hear.

During the hearing aid review sessions, once the aids and ears have been checked and progress discussed, the clinician will want to cycle through aided and unaided measurements. Both are important. The unaided measurements give a clearer picture of the extent of the loss and help us to fine-tune the hearing aids. The aided measurements can be used to find out what use the child is able to make of his aided hearing and to explore his dynamic range (the difference between what he can just hear and what he can just tolerate). It is important also to explore which speech sounds are reaching the child. This can be checked at this age by substituting speech sounds for the whistles and noises we commonly use. Presenting the Ling sounds (Ling, 1989; see also Chapter 8), or even just talking to the child, can give a useful indicator of hearing for speech.

Hearing aid reviews cycle round and round this process, constantly checking and tuning the aids, perhaps changing them completely as the picture continues to build, and thus giving the child the best chance of making full use of his aided hearing.

Insert phones (see Chapter 1) are particularly useful at this stage. Most loudspeaker systems will only produce sounds up to 90 dB. This may not be enough to reach more severely impaired children. Because they are not hearing the sounds, they do not show responses, which is very frustrating for the parents and clinician. Insert phones can reach up to 120 dB. Most children will respond at this level, even if only to low frequencies, where they feel, rather than hear, the sound. Suddenly then, the child begins to show clear signs of reacting to sounds. This is rewarding in itself and also confirms that the lack of response to the loudspeaker sounds was probably because the sounds were simply not loud enough rather than because the child was incapable of responding.

'So I just sit there and watch?'

Parents are not passive bystanders in the process. Habilitation is a process in which parents take a leading role, and this should always be made clear to them. They can bring vital information about the use and benefits of the hearing aids at home. They may also have their own strong views about what information they themselves want. For example, a family may be quite happy to watch the aided thresholds being measured but find it much more difficult to observe unaided testing as this brings home to them, every time it is done, the fact and the extent of their child's disability. Any hearing aid review should therefore proceed along a path agreed by both parents and clinician, and the choice of path will form part of the discussion at the start of each review.

Sometimes parents can be involved in the actual testing, although this does not always work well. Children may perform less co-operatively with parents than with clinicians, although parents are often excellent sources of advice and inspiration when the session is grinding to a halt through lack of child co-operation – after all, they know their child better than anyone. It is useful to encourage both parents to come to the hearing aid review. In that way, both are involved in the process and can share the responsibility of helping their child. Furthermore, it gives one parent the opportunity to observe the session without being directly involved, by sitting with the tester, while the other remains with the child. Parents say that they get a very different view in this situation, and they can sometimes see responses that are not otherwise as easy to see.

Finally, parents can find it useful to be updated briefly as the session proceeds. It is their child the clinician is doing things to, and it is reassuring for them to know what is going on. This is particularly true if insert phones are being used as the parents cannot hear what level of sound is being delivered. The updating can be delivered without disrupting the flow of the session, but this takes practice.

Summary

This chapter has discussed some of the challenges that are presented by aiding very young hearing impaired children. It has dealt with the problem of introducing parents and their child to hearing aids, of selecting and tuning the aids, often based at first on limited information, of helping the child adjust to the aid and of exploring the benefits it gives him. It is a complex process that unfolds over time, with parents and professionals working in close and equal partnership.

References

Adams JW (1991) You and Your Hearing-impaired Child. Washington, DC: Clerc Books, Gallaudet University Press.

Archbold S (1997) Cochlear implants. In McCracken W, Laoide-Kemp S (Eds) Audiology in Education. London: Whurr.

Brett R, Joshua A (1997) Earmoulds. In McCracken W, Laoide-Kemp S (Eds) Audiology in Education. London: Whurr.

Byrne D (1983) Theoretical prescriptive approaches to selecting the gain and frequency response of a hearing aid. Monographs in Contemporary Audiology 4: 1.

Byrne D, Dillon H (1986) The National Acoustic Laboratories' (NAL) new procedure for selecting the gain and frequency response of a hearing aid. Ear and Hearing 7: 257–65.

Green RJ (1993) Hearing aid selection and evaluation in pre-school children. In McCormick B (Ed.) Paediatric Audiology 0–5 Years, 2nd Edn. London: Whurr.

Ling D (1989) Foundations of Spoken Language for Hearing-Impaired Children. Washington, DC: AG Bell Association for the Deaf.

National Deaf Children's Society (1992) Cochlear Implants and Deaf Children. London: NDCS.

National Deaf Children's Society (1994) Quality Standards in Paediatric Audiology, Vol. I: Guidelines for the Early Identification of Hearing Impairment. London: NDCS.

National Deaf Children's Society (1996) Quality Standards in Paediatric Audiology, Vol II: The Audiological Management of the Child with Permanent Hearing Loss. London: NDCS.

Seewald RC (1992) The desired sensation level method for fitting children: version 3. Hearing Journal 45(4): 36–41.

Chapter 4
Children with mild and moderate hearing losses

ROGER WILLS

The diagnosis of hearing loss, particularly permanent hearing loss in a child, is always a complex and distressing affair. This is especially true for the parents, who usually have had no previous knowledge or contact with hearing loss in their past.

When the hearing loss is severe or profound, there will often have been an earlier period when one or both parents thought that something was wrong. They may have suspected a hearing problem, although they are naturally likely to have hoped to be proved wrong, or at least to have hoped that the condition would not be permanent. Severe or profound hearing loss is likely to have become evident at an early stage since the perceptive parent, or other carer, will have begun to notice a lack of typical reaction on the part of the child to normal conversation or household sounds. The situation is very different for the child with a mild or moderate loss, who may reach the age of 2 or 3 before his hearing impairment is diagnosed.

The contrast between the severely deaf child and the child with a mild-to-moderate hearing loss can lead to much confusion in the minds of the parents and the extended family. The relatively clear lack of auditory awareness on the part of the severely deaf child is distressing and likely to lead to an early appeal for help. However, the confusing and apparently contradictory picture with a mild or moderate hearing loss will often delay any formal investigation of the child's behaviour. The child with this small degree of hearing loss will not be behaving in ways that many lay people regard as typical of their understanding of deafness. The common perception of hearing loss or deafness is that it is always severe, leaving the sufferer plainly unable to hear anything at all. Playgroup leaders, nursery teachers, childminders and others can be forgiven for not realizing that hearing loss can be of any degree: the mild or moderately deaf child is not deaf enough to alert them to the possibility of a hearing loss (Candlish, 1996).

When the hearing loss is finally confirmed, it may be as a result of a screening check secondary to the investigation of a speech and language delay, or an apparent behaviour problem, rather than specifically on the suspicion of a hearing loss. This situation can give rise to major problems of acceptance and constructive action on the part of the parents, who will need sensitive support. If the hearing loss is described by those involved in the diagnosis as mild or moderate, these terms may serve to suggest that the loss is not very significant. 'Mild', 'moderate', 'severe' and 'profound', as descriptors for degrees of hearing loss, are a useful shorthand for audiologists and teachers of the deaf when discussing these issues. However, the terms cannot be regarded as reflecting the degree of handicap that the loss will cause. Even a mild hearing loss is recognized to cause a significant difficulty in terms of speech and language development, and educational progress.

How can hearing loss be missed?

Very few people in general associate permanent hearing loss with children. In common experience, hearing loss, more usually referred to by most people as deafness, is associated with adults, especially the elderly. It comes as a considerable surprise to most parents to learn that, in a typical health district of 500 000 people, there may be 300 children wearing hearing aids, although they may not express surprise that there could be 30 000 adults with hearing aids in the same area. Over half of these children will have a mild or moderate hearing loss, and will form a large part of the caseload of every audiology and special education service (Davies et al., 1997).

It useful to consider the ways in which a mild or moderate hearing loss in small children may be masked by other factors associated with parent–infant interaction, glue ear and changes in the child's behaviour.

Parent–infant interaction

Much of the parental interaction occurs at quite close range during the baby's early months. The parent or carer may seldom be more than 1 metre away from the child when going about all the usual tasks that make up his care. A great deal of the time, the child will be held by the carer, who will be talking and interacting with the child using normal conversational levels of voice. When playing or singing, the carer will probably be using even higher levels of voice. Many speech sounds at a distance of around 30 cm are at a loudness of around 70 dBA, so that even if the child has a mild or moderate hearing loss, the sound levels will still be enough to make the voice interesting and stimulating. The close proximity of the parent to a child with a mild or moderate hearing loss will to this extent mask the presence of the hearing loss.

Later, the child becomes more mobile, and common distances between child and carer become more variable. Now the hearing loss may make clear hearing unreliable at a distance, but the child will continue to hear well enough when close to. The picture can become further complicated by other factors. With growing familiarity with the household and care routines, the child will be learning to anticipate the demands of the carers. The child appears to follow a command or co-operates with a request, but it is not clear how the communication occurred. Was it hearing or familiarity with the routine that led the child to behave as required?

Similarly, the small hearing impaired child in a family setting with older normally hearing siblings will learn to take clues from them about the demands of home life. On occasions, the older children intuitively take on the role of compensating for the hearing difficulties of the smaller child. They may interpret the small child's poor speech or reinforce at closer range the conversation of the parent who is further away. The apparently reasonable notion that the child can hear when necessary, or 'when he wants to', can lead to a reluctance to regard the variable behaviour as needing a medical opinion. Only later, when direct interaction occurs with children of the same age, perhaps at nursery or playgroup, will the child stand out as being different from the others. Even at this stage, there are often plausible reasons to reject the idea that anything significant may be amiss.

Let us take a look at the case of Adam.

Case history

Adam was aged 4 years and 3 months when he was referred by the family doctor to a speech and language therapist. He was described as wary of strangers and varying between shy and energetically disruptive when among other children. He seemed to be having tantrums over his inability to communicate with other children and adults. His vocabulary was considerable, but much of it was unclear except to his family. Adam attended playgroup and would soon be going to school as a 'rising 5', but the playgroup staff were nervous of his unpredictable behaviour with other children.

The speech therapist saw him three times before referring him on to a developmental language clinic since she suspected a specific language disorder rather than straightforward delay. Adam attended the clinic four times, seeing paediatricians and speech therapists, before one of the speech therapists there asked whether his hearing had been tested. He was now 5 years and 4 months old. In the audiology department, Adam co-operated with puretone audiometry and demonstrated a moderate bilateral sensorineural hearing loss, with hearing thresholds of 35 dBHL up to 1000 Hz, and down to 55 dBHL at 4000 Hz. Within a week, he was fitted with postaural hearing aids and was referred on to a speech therapist specializing in work with hearing impaired children.

In the 2 years since the original diagnosis and hearing aid fitting, Adam's hearing has become a little worse, but he has made great progress with his language skills and attends a resourced unit for hearing impaired children in a mainstream infant school. He no longer has any abnormal or difficult behaviour and has made many friends in school. His parents have come to terms with the overall situation and are very positive in support of Adam and his continuing progress.

Much can be learned from stories like that of Adam, and at every stage parents, educationalists and health-care professionals would do well to routinely consider the possibility of hearing loss when they are assessing children.

Glue ear

Most parents are aware that, during the infant years, many children suffer variable hearing through the common problems associated with middle ear disorders. They may know the condition as glue ear rather than otitis media with effusion (OME), but they are aware that it occurs. These hearing losses are referred to as conductive and are usually temporary, rather than sensorineural and permanent. Parents do not consider anything to be unduly troubling when the small child appears not to hear well during or following a cold or respiratory disorder. Some small children get prolonged periods of such disorders, especially during the winter months, and especially during the period when they first begin to mix with other small children at nursery or playgroup. The child may be under the care of the family doctor for these problems and even perhaps for known problems of acute otitis media. The inconsolable, screaming child with earache in the small hours of the night will have disrupted the whole family.

The hearing problems caused in this way, or in the case of a child with a mild or moderate sensorineural hearing loss made worse by the condition, will not cause undue concern. The cause will be thought to be self-evident. The child has earache and glue ear, and is seeing the doctor. 'Of course he cannot hear well at the moment,' the parent might say, 'but he will be all right when his ears are better.' It is not surprising that parents do not think of the possibility of a permanent hearing loss combined with the OME. However, it is often this combined disorder that so confuses the early diagnosis of mild or moderate sensorineural hearing loss. The common middle ear problem does not cause great alarm, the hearing loss is regarded as a routine matter, certainly temporary, and the whole problem may not be taken seriously enough.

If the OME persists, the child may be referred to the hospital to see the ENT consultant. Part of the diagnostic process is likely to involve conduction of hearing tests by the audiologists in the department. The child who has underlying hearing that is normal will only be likely to show a mild conductive hearing loss caused by the middle ear condition. In contrast, the child who has an underlying sensorineural hearing loss will show an accumulated hearing loss from the two causes. This 'double' hearing loss will be greater than that commonly associated with OME alone. At this point, it will become clear to the audiologists and the ENT specialist that the resolution of this child's problem is a more urgent matter than the routine case. This is especially true when there is an accompanying history of speech and language delay or difficulty.

Even before the onset of the otitis media, the parents may have recognized the child as slow to progress with speech and language. It may have been noticed that the child was unable to learn the correct words to rhymes or songs used at playgroup or school. The strange or invented version that the child thinks to be correct may be thought of as rather funny and appealing within the family, little recognizing that the underlying cause could be a sensorineural hearing problem.

Where the middle ear problem resolves or does not provoke a referral to the hospital, the delay in the detection of the underlying sensorineural hearing loss continues. Eventually, as in the case of Adam, it may be the continuing speech and language delay that finally provokes referral, although not necessarily to an ENT or audiology department. This situation, in which the child's problems are regarded as connected at first with speech and language development, and then later also with hearing impairment, which may or nor be permanent, can be confusing and difficult for parents to understand. High-frequency sensorineural hearing loss, with good hearing for low frequencies but poor hearing for higher frequencies, is also difficult for lay people to comprehend. If a child is clearly hearing many sounds quite normally, parents and others will find the suggestion of a hearing loss very hard to accept. Yet it is very common for sensorineural hearing loss to affect the hearing for some sounds more than others.

Changes in behaviour

Hearing loss of any degree, including that in the child with only a mild or moderate degree of hearing loss, is likely to enhance the visual awareness of the child as an unconscious compensatory mechanism. The skill may extend to a rudimentary ability to lip-read and often to greater sensitivity than usual to clues from body language and natural gesture. In the case of some children who have a severe degree of hearing loss, there is often such a remarkable visual awareness of their surroundings that they are not at all straightforward to test where there may be any visual clue to the test sounds. This is especially true for hearing tests carried out in the child's home. Moving shadows, perfume and reflections in ornaments can all give tiny clues that lead a child apparently to react to the test sound. It may only be in the specialized audiology test room that it becomes possible to ensure that only the hearing is being tested! Even then, the anxious parent or grandparent can give inadvertent clues to the visually aware child if the audiologist is not vigilant.

Additional factors may also serve to confuse when piecing together the picture of the behaviour of a small hearing impaired child. Equally, some of these factors can alert the clinician to the possibility of hearing loss. Tantrums that could be caused by communication frustration rather than, for example, common sibling rivalry are a helpful index to the degree of language inadequacy that a child may be experiencing. Allied to this is the reputation of some small children to be unable to play well with other children, or to be disruptive in a group. It is not difficult to believe that a small child unable to follow the rules of a group activity that relies on hearing the spoken word may become resentful and disruptive, and then unpopular with the group.

Similarly, the child who hears reasonably only at close range will appear erratic, unco-operative, even ill mannered and disobedient to those who are unaware of the hearing problem. Naturally, the child who is genuinely unco-operative and mischievous in addition to having a genuine hearing loss will tax the patience of any carer. These reputations, once established, are difficult to reverse since they tend to be noted and passed on to new carers meeting the child for the first time. Other close-range hearing situations may also serve to confuse. The child may be noted to sit close to the television but to enjoy watching, and therefore apparently to be hearing adequately. However, programming for the very young is cleverly designed to be highly visually attractive, dependent for example upon visual humour, and will usually hold the attention of most small children even if there is no dialogue or if the dialogue is not in their own language.

In the case of the hearing impaired child who has OME as well, there are some other side-effects of the OME that may also serve to complicate the overall picture further. OME sometimes causes a reduced tolerance to loud noise, so-called hyperacusis. This will be recognized as an extreme reaction, even terror, at the sound of low-flying aircraft or fire engine sirens, for example. Hyperacusis may be noticed to be a greater problem when the OME is worse. This behaviour might be thought eccentric in a child previously interested in aircraft but should be seen as not uncommon with OME. Similarly, some children experience variable vestibular or balance disturbances with OME. The child who has evidence of frequent falls and accidents, and who is described as clumsy or having poor balance, unable to dispense with bicycle stabilizers for example, may be affected by the middle ear effusion. This situation may complicate judgements made by paediatricians when assessing developmental issues that relate to independent mobility, motor control and allied matters.

In a similar way, a child might be regarded as having a degree of learning difficulty rather than a hearing loss, when in fact the hearing problem may be wholly or partly responsible for aspects of developmental delay. These judgements can be fraught with danger since, paradoxically, some parents of children with genuine developmental delay and mild learning difficulties may prefer to suggest that the child has a simple hearing impairment. Despite the distress and problems for most parents of accepting the presence of a hearing loss in their child, there are those who find this a more acceptable and preferable cause for the child's problems than the diagnosis of a learning difficulty.

Confirmation of a permanent hearing loss

When the decision is taken to investigate for the possibility of hearing loss, the outcome will depend to an extent upon the quality of the referral and the referral route chosen for the child. Often because of the difficulty of testing such children in a domestic setting, there will have been uncertainty about the validity of any hearing tests carried out in the home by the health visitor or nurse working from the family doctor's surgery. These uncertainties usually reflect the unsatisfactory test environment rather than the skill of the personnel. The health visitor may have been uncertain, or the parents may have expressed concern, so that the test may have been repeated a number of times. Alternatively, the child with a mild or moderate hearing loss may have been 'passed' as normal since he will clearly react to a great deal of sound if not to the very quietest levels. Even at the low sound levels, the child may have reacted, for example to some visual clue, and been regarded as within normal limits for hearing.

The parents may also be unwilling to contemplate the possibility of hearing loss. This can result from the perception that hearing loss or deafness is inevitably always severe, yet the child can clearly react and respond to many sounds. The child may be regarded as wilful and able to hear when he wants to. Delays commonly occur at this stage, so it may only be later, with growing concern about speech and language abilities, that the matter is raised again.

Notwithstanding any other disabilities, medical conditions or developmental problems that the child may have, it is important whenever doubt exists that hearing is investigated at the earliest opportunity, in a well-resourced and experienced specialist paediatric audiology department. Such departments will have close links with the ENT department and with other departments to which secondary referrals may become necessary. It is established good practice to refer children diagnosed as permanently hearing impaired on to departments of ophthalmology, developmental paediatrics and, where appropriate, genetics. These referrals will ensure that the fullest possible understanding of the child's needs, and all the necessary advice, counselling and support can be given to the parents.

The gathering of evidence to build up a full picture of the complete circumstances surrounding the child and the hearing loss is necessary to identify the detail of the child's subsequent support requirements. The specialist team from the education authority whose job it is to support hearing impaired children in the education system will need information from this collection of evidence. With their help, the parents will be made aware of the options for educational placement and be helped to understand the rights of parents and children under the terms of the current legislation covering special education. In the UK, a Statement of Special Educational Need may be recommended, compiled from the accumulated evidence gathered when the hearing loss is investigated. This Statement ensures that the need for any unusual or specialized educational provision and supervision will be identified and provided (see Chapter 7).

The diagnostic process

When the child is seen in an audiology department, there will be two stages to the diagnostic process. First is the assessment of the child's hearing and then, if a hearing loss is found, an assessment of the probable cause or causes of the disorder.

As we have seen, the child with a mild or moderate hearing loss typically does not cause concern when very young. As a result, the child is usually old enough for hearing testing by visual reinforcement audiometry (VRA). With this technique, the child is distracted from minimal play by test sounds made in the room. The sounds are initially accompanied by a visual reinforcement or reward such as an animated toy, but when the child has come to expect this, the sound is played without the visual reward. Once the child is seen to react to the sound, the visual reward is given as well. Conditioning a small child to react to VRA is usually quite quick, and the test is recognized as accurate and powerful in these circumstances. However, it is not a test in which the child is actively listening for the test sounds since he is being distracted from an alternative activity and is not of an age at which the notion of attending to a listening task is realistic. VRA can be used successfully from as little as 7 or 8 months of age with children who are functioning normally from the developmental point of view and who are without significant visual handicap.

Variations of the VRA technique can be used with children who do have developmental or visual problems. Other techniques, such as traditional distraction testing, may be equally valid if used with care, although the relative lack of precision in quantifying the loudness of the stimulus sounds used during distraction testing can impair the quality of the results obtained.

In a sound-treated test room with appropriately chosen and calibrated test sounds, these sound field test procedures can yield very accurate and repeatable results. In the few minutes of co-operation and interest that may be available with a small child, it is usually possible to screen for the hearing levels of the main sounds used in speech. The tests will not necessarily give good information about how one ear compares with the other, although this may be considered less crucial than showing at least one ear to be hearing to within normal limits. When it is important to measure the hearing levels in each ear separately, it is possible to conduct tests such as VRA using insert earphones rather than a loudspeaker system.

From around 3 years old, most children will be quite capable of co-operative test procedures. In these, the child will be listening for the test sounds and responding with some simple repetitive game or play task each time a sound is heard. These tests are qualitatively better than VRA since the child is now more likely to be relatively still and listening for the sounds. It is not unusual for some children to manage these tests at an even earlier age, and the progression on to tests that can give separate results for each ear becomes possible. Headphones or insert earphones will allow the testing of each ear separately, although the test will, of course, take longer than for binaural listening in the sound field room. The child's attention span and familiarity with the test situation and the audiology staff, as well as the skill of the audiologist, will determine just how much testing can be done at any one appointment.

If the child is not found to be responding at normal hearing levels, a judgement must made on whether this is a valid and repeatable result. Small children may give variable reactions to the test sounds: they may be either very nervous in the test room or over-excited and anxious to please. When the result is felt to be consistent and repeatable, and reliably indicates hearing below normal levels, the involvement of an ENT specialist becomes necessary. This doctor will investigate the many possible causes of hearing loss and the possibility of medical or surgical treatment. Naturally, with this age group, the possibility of the hearing loss being caused or made worse by simple OME will be examined. Simple screening devices for the likelihood of OME use techniques of tympanometry or reflectometry to indicate the possibility of middle ear effusion. These devices, which resemble the otoscope commonly used for looking into the ear, allow the monitoring of middle ear effusion and, by implication, Eustachian tube function. The test is very quick, taking only a few seconds to record a result, and although the suspicious small child may wriggle and render the test impossible, the procedure is in no way painful or even uncomfortable.

When the hearing loss is found to be conductive, i.e. the problem is in the outer or middle ear and interferes with the transfer of sound to the inner ear, this does not mean that it is necessarily caused by OME. There are some congenital conditions in which there may be structural middle ear abnormalities quite unnoticeable externally. Congenital conductive hearing loss is not necessarily curable either surgically or medically. Where there may be thought to be a correctable structural middle ear problem, it is not likely that surgery will be contemplated until the child is older. With growth, the operation site becomes larger and the surgery technically more feasible. Surgeons are reluctant to offer any intervention that could impose a significant risk of making the problem worse.

'Double' hearing loss

A 'double' hearing loss describes the situation in which OME is present in addition to a mild or moderate sensorineural hearing loss. In these cases, where the hearing loss is greater than that commonly associated with OME alone, it is important to resolve the OME as a matter of urgency. This is especially true when the hearing loss is found to be clearly moderate and bordering on the severe or worse. When the simple treatable part of the problem has been dealt with, it is possible properly to assess the child's hearing.

The routine clinical approach to the diagnosis of OME causing only a mild hearing loss, i.e. not a 'double' hearing loss, would usually be one of 'watchful waiting' – the child is merely monitored during the period when the condition would normally resolve. OME is self-limiting in the sense that the condition usually resolves spontaneously. Unfortunately, this process could be prolonged, especially in the winter months, when colds, coughs and respiratory problems, which often lead to OME, are common. However, in the case of a disproportionate degree of hearing loss, all available 'short cuts' to resolve the OME are appropriate. This may justify an admission into hospital for myringotomy and grommet insertion as soon as possible.

If the behaviour of the child in the test room, or the complication of additional problems such as developmental delay or learning difficulties, makes any hearing testing problematic or very difficult, there are likely also to be difficulties with achieving an adequate ENT examination. Where there is strong evidence of the likelihood of OME, it may be felt appropriate to admit the child for an ENT examination under anaesthetic, followed by whatever surgery is found to be justified. This may include myringotomy and the insertion of grommets, and perhaps adenoidectomy to reduce the likelihood of the recurrence of OME. In addition, it is possible to carry out specialized hearing tests under the anaesthetic once the ears have been examined and any middle ear fluid removed. Brainstem electrical response audiometry, or auditory brainstem response tests, can reliably show the hearing thresholds for the middle-to-high-frequency sounds, and variations of these techniques can give good information about hearing over a wider range of frequencies (see Chapter 1). If a hearing loss is found despite the absence of middle ear fluid, the probability is that it is indeed sensorineural. Occasionally, the results from tests carried out within minutes of myringotomy are subsequently found to have been pessimistic, but this is not common.

Where the hearing loss is significant and the co-operation of the child when awake is in doubt, a further advantage of the anaesthetic can be in taking impressions of the ears for the manufacture of hearing aid earmoulds. Naturally, the parents should have been counselled beforehand to be aware of this possible outcome. It is unusual for there to be a great problem repeating the impressions in due course with the child awake since by that time the child will have become more accustomed to ear examination and the use of hearing aids and earmoulds. In the case of mild or moderate hearing loss, most children will be fitted with behind-the-ear hearing aids. These aids come in an enormous range of performance and ergonomic variations, and will usually provide very good amplification for these degrees of hearing loss (see Chapter 3). In addition, it is likely that, in co-operation with the specialist supporting team from the education authority, the aids will be chosen in anticipation of the need for direct audio input being required at some later stage.

This hospital admission should be followed up quite quickly by an outpatient attendance for confirmation that the grommets are in place and working, and for further behavioural hearing tests to measure the hearing again. There will often be good evidence from the family of improved hearing at home, together with evidence of the advantages of adenoidectomy when this has been done. Where there is still a hearing loss, of a lesser degree than previously but probably now confirmed as sensorineural, it becomes appropriate to investigate more fully the cause of the hearing loss. It will thus be necessary to arrange secondary referrals to other types of medical opinion. For example, it is necessary to confirm that the general development of the child is age appropriate, that there are no undiagnosed visual difficulties and that any genetic implications of the hearing disorder will be investigated. When there is a collection of features thought to be a known syndrome affecting children, it becomes necessary to confirm this possibility and counsel the family accordingly (see Chapter 2).

Permanent conductive hearing loss

Permanent hearing loss may not be sensorineural in origin. Hearing loss caused by prolonged or repeated infections can cause irreversible damage in the ear, or the ear may be damaged by injury. Some children will have had so many episodes of acute OME that there may have been a number of admissions to hospital for myringotomy and grommets, or long-stay tympanostomy tubes (T tubes), during their infant years. Some of these children never recover good middle ear function and may remain with some conductive hearing loss even after they have ceased to get middle ear infections. The eardrum may show signs of past troubles with scarring, as well as white patches known as tympanosclerosis, which betray the past infective process. The remaining hearing loss may have a sensorineural element as well, so that the bone conduction hearing is not good either. In extreme cases, where the eardrums have become permanently retracted, there will be a risk of further problems developing, and there will be a need for continuing ENT care.

Perforated eardrums as a consequence of injury or infection may be treated surgically with grafts to repair the perforation, but improved hearing is not a foregone conclusion in these cases. It may be helpful to make the ear clinically safer from further infection, but the hearing may still be abnormal. Where a significant hearing loss remains, even though it may be conductive, it may be justifiable to move on to hearing aid provision. Parents are likely to be disappointed that, after all they and the child have been through in terms of surgery and treatment, the child's hearing is still not good. It is worth remembering that these children are probably among the very small minority who, before the advent of antibiotics and modern ENT medical and surgical techniques, would have been at risk of meningitis or cerebral abscess. Indeed, in the 1920s, infant death from these causes was not at all uncommon. To come through all this nowadays with an outcome no worse than a hearing loss can justifiably be seen as a relief.

Accepting the hearing loss

The diagnostic and treatment process so far may have served to reduce the hearing loss to some degree, but there may be the new problem of convincing the parents that, even with the improved hearing, there is still the need to continue on to hearing aid fitting. The previous moderate-bordering-on-severe hearing loss may now be a mild-bordering-on-moderate hearing loss, but it will still be a real disadvantage to the child in a classroom setting. The parents' recent experience is, however, of improved hearing at home. The use of the sound field test room is very helpful in these circumstances. Despite the fact that the child may be quite capable of headphone audiometry, the overriding disadvantage for the parents is that they do not hear for themselves any direct evidence of the degree of hearing loss. Assuming that one or both parents has good hearing, the tactic of testing the child in the sound field test room is extremely helpful for them. They will hear for themselves the point at which the child ceases to respond to the test sounds.

Additional tests in the sound field room showing the ability to discriminate speech accurately will further help them to understand the crucial difference between hearing with difficulty and hearing at lower sound levels with good confidence. It is then much more straightforward to explain the importance of this in the context of the classroom listening situation. The analogy of being able to see without reading glasses, but only to see well with them, is appropriate.

Once it is clear that the hearing loss is sensorineural, permanent mixed or permanent conductive in character, prompt decisions about hearing aid provision are important. It is not entirely appropriate to generalize, but, as a rule of thumb, it can be said that when the majority of thresholds on a pure tone audiogram are worse than 30 dBHL, a mild hearing loss, it is likely that hearing aids will be beneficial. Obviously, with the mildest of hearing losses, hearing aids will be appropriate only in selected circumstances. In most school lessons, the hearing aids will certainly be important, as they will be at other times when valuable language opportunities arise. However, the hearing aids will not be as useful in noisy places or when the child is involved in tough physical sport or play.

The audiologists will have set up the hearing aid system to avoid the likelihood of discomfort from loud noise when the aids are in use. However, the electronics in the hearing aids, in suppressing the worst effects of high sound inputs to the aids, may cause some distortion, which can reduce the benefit of the aids in these circumstances. In addition, it is a common feature of most hearing losses that the hearing system in the ear and the brain has a reduced ability to select speech from competing noise. This problem is caused by the changes within the hearing mechanism that caused the hearing loss, especially within the organ of hearing, the cochlea (Moore, 1995). Some hearing losses and some hearing aid technologies are better than others in these respects. Parents and other carers must be counselled towards a realistic understanding of hearing aid benefits and limitations.

Hearing aid benefit and management

When the hearing aids are fitted, it becomes possible to use the test room to demonstrate the difference in hearing ability when aided. This kind of unaided versus aided comparison helps the audiologist too, of course, but much of it is especially important for the parents. They have to justify the whole process at home and to the extended family and friends who may well share their initial scepticism. Sometimes there are real problems for the parents in agreeing with both the diagnosis and the action that has followed. Equally, in order to gain acceptance and constructive support from the whole family, some of whom may share the childcare, it is necessary that all concerned become convinced about the situation. Occasionally, there is firm denial, even aggressive protest, from other family members at the suggestion of any genetic or family-related connection with the occurrence of the hearing loss. Where the hearing loss is clearly severe or profound, there may be similar feelings, but since the hearing loss is so much more evident, there is seldom a denial of the presence of the hearing loss.

It is usually the wish of the audiologists that the hearing aids are in use for the majority of the day, but this may not occur in practice. It is often the convenient perception of the family that the hearing aids are for use in school only. This may be a lingering effect of the belief that the child appears to hear adequately at home, or there may be reluctance on the part of the child to co-operate with hearing aid use out of school. Children who claim that the hearing aid is uncomfortable will often add to the insecurity of parents' reluctance to push for hearing aid use in case the discomfort is real. There may also be real or perceived unhelpful reactions from the child's peer group. Alternatively, there may be some genuine concern on the part of the parents about the safety and security of the hearing aids when used during play.

There are real issues of common sense concerning the use of the hearing aids during activities in which there is a high probability of damage or loss of the aids but in which communication is not a major problem. At one extreme, the aids are obviously not to be used for swimming, but in terms of other sports and play activities, the best policy may be much less obvious. There do need to be ground rules for the safety of the hearing aids, but there should also be an attempt to maximize use of the aids within those constraints. However, it is important to strike a balance between natural caution and the need for the child to be hearing natural language as consistently as possible. The philosophy of the audiology department with respect to the occasional damage and loss of hearing aids is important here. To some extent, the parent of a small child who never experiences one of these problems is probably not really trying! It is very difficult to get hearing aids used consistently in small children who do not yet understand concepts such as 'fragile' and 'expensive' without any damage ever occurring. Audiology departments must budget for all of the predictable running costs of the paediatric hearing aid programme. Most parents are genuinely upset by the damage or loss of a hearing aid and will go to great lengths to retrieve it. A mother recently told how she had moved every piece of wood from a log pile in the garden where her small son had been at a birthday party. Another child had 'allegedly' removed the hearing aids from her son and thrown them into the pile. She single-handedly moved over a tonne of wood in her efforts to find the lost aids. The aids were not in the log pile but were finally found elsewhere in the garden.

However, repeated damage to, loss of or blatant vandalism to hearing aids does raise justifiable questions about the adequacy of care and home management of the hearing aid system. Some hearing aids will be in use by the children of families in poor social circumstances, where it is unrealistic to expect ideal home management and where severe sanctions for damage or losses are completely inappropriate. There is an overriding need to maintain a constructive relationship with the families of children with hearing aids even when the management of the hearing aids is poor.

Some hearing aid manufacturers provide care kits for the management of the hearing aid system. These kits are cleverly designed to be appealing to small children and to help parents to manage the care of the aids at home. Accessories such as attractive hearing aid stickers, colouring books and soft toys can add an atmosphere of fun rather than disappointment to hearing aid use. The pride and novelty associated with the presentation of the care kit promotes a good attitude towards the hearing aid system on the part of the child and the family.

Where children are allowed, even encouraged, by parents not to use the aids out of school, the language competence of the child is likely to suffer significantly. In addition, the familiarity with the hearing aids and with hearing aid listening will suffer during school holiday periods. Hearing aids may or may not be maintained adequately in these circumstances, and it is less likely that the earmoulds will be kept up to date in terms of fit if they are only intermittently used. In order to avoid these problems, it is necessary to be clear about the expectation of the pattern of hearing aid use from the time when it becomes evident that aids are needed. With the infant-age child, many of these problems are more manageable, but consistent hearing aid use later can be a problem.

Hearing aid benefit will be reduced by high levels of background noise and also in rooms or buildings with poor acoustics. It is crucial that the supporting team from the special education services of the education authority is involved from the beginning, when hearing aid fitting is planned with children. Their help is needed for good liaison, support and guidance for the classroom teachers when a child in mainstream school is to be fitted with hearing aids. There may be an understandable perception on the part of school teachers that, once fitted with hearing aids, the child can be treated as if normally hearing. This simplistic misconception is shared by many adults who are fitted with hearing aids. They, too, are often surprised to find that their hearing is anything other than completely normal once aided. There will need to be changes of teaching style when a hearing aid user is among a class of children, even where the hearing loss is mild. In addition, with small children, the class teacher may need to share responsibility for aspects of hearing aid management.

Where the hearing loss is in the moderate category, the need for hearing aid fitting is even more obvious. Hearing aid use will be justified for a greater proportion of the time. However, it remains the case that these children with mild and moderate hearing losses may be perceived by the parents and families as coping perfectly well unaided at home. This complacency is an error of judgement, one seldom made with any real appreciation of the disadvantage that the child will suffer. It is true, up to a point, that the child may function with less obvious difficulty at home, for the same reasons that may have caused the diagnosis of the hearing loss to have been delayed in the first place. However, now that the hearing loss is confirmed, it is important to maximize the child's exposure to natural language and vocabulary. At home, the child might appear able to hear adequately without the aids, but even here he will miss useful linguistic experience and language learning opportunities without the hearing aids in place. Conversation is a fluid and variable experience; at any moment, new vocabulary or linguistic variations can occur that would benefit the child. Without the hearing aids enhancing the opportunity to absorb these experiences, the child's ability, progress and confidence is threatened.

In order that hearing aids can be effectively used at home, it is necessary that families understand that they may need to 'regulate' household noise. It is certainly not helpful for parents to insist on hearing aid use at home and then take no care to limit meaningless, even uncomfortable, background noise. Permanent music and the sound of household appliances will leave the hearing aid-using child in hopeless confusion. It is not difficult to make small changes to routines at home so that, when important conversation and language opportunities are available, the background noise is kept to a minimum. A routine in which the hearing aids are in use at home for part of every day is to be preferred. It is reasonable for this experience to be planned so that it is pleasurable for the child.

In the special listening situation of the normal mainstream classroom, the child with hearing aids will not hear as well as other children, even when using the hearing aids. This problem occurs because the room is larger than a typical room at home, the acoustics may not be ideal, and there is usually a constant level of competing noise. The teaching style adopted by the class teacher will affect the noise level, but even a well-behaved but busy class of children can be expected to generate a significant buzz of activity. Knowing that impaired hearing is likely to have poor selectivity for speech in noise, it is necessary to find a solution to this problem.

Hearing aids fitted to children usually have a means of connection for a direct input from a personal radio system. These systems, generally supplied by the special education services, allow the child to hear the most important sound, that of the teacher's voice, with very good clarity. The radio transmitter, about the size of an audio-cassette tape, is worn by the teacher, with a microphone clipped on to clothing not very far from the mouth. The radio receiver, of similar size, is worn by the child and connected directly to the hearing aids. The system ensures that the teacher's voice will always be audible to the child above the classroom noise (see Chapter 3). The special education team will help the mainstream teacher to learn to use this equipment effectively, both within the classroom and outside. The range of transmission may be as great as 200 metres, which can be very useful in the playground! This type of supplementary equipment, and the liaison between the audiology department and the special education services, should ensure that hearing impaired children in a mainstream school setting can be expected to achieve their educational potential.

Regular review of children with hearing aids

Even when hearing aid use is well established, and school circumstances are under good control, there will be a need to continue to monitor the hearing and the hearing aid system. Sadly, many sensorineural hearing losses do prove to be degenerative. In some ways, this situation should not cause more alarm than the predictable slow change in the prescription one might expect if a child uses glasses. However, since the experience of hearing loss in children is so much less familiar to most parents, the concept that the hearing loss may become worse with time is likely to cause a greater level of concern. Small children will probably be seen for periodic review by the audiology department at intervals of not longer than 2 or 3 months. The earmoulds may not fit for much longer than this, and the hearing aids will often need maintenance since they are subject to much 'wear and tear' when used by small children.

Typically, these regular reviews will include checking the ears, the hearing, the hearing aid system and the aided hearing levels. With the pre-school and infant school-age groups, there is the need to monitor for OME, and it is always necessary to monitor the hearing for possible change. It may also be that the child is continuing to see the ENT doctor for regular review, especially if there is OME or grommets are perhaps in place.

In addition, there is likely to be the need for periodic dewaxing of the ear canals. When hearing aids are in use, the wax tends to accumulate in the ear canal at the point where the earmould ends. This will eventually interfere with hearing aid performance and may cause acoustic feedback whistling. As new earmoulds become necessary with the growth of the child, regular impressions for new earmoulds will be needed, but this may not be safe if there is an accumulation of wax. Most children become used to the dewaxing procedure and will co-operate well, but some will need considerable encouragement to learn to trust those involved. Where the wax is hard and might be uncomfortable to remove, the doctor will usually recommend drops to soften the wax first. It is essential that the ENT doctors recognize the importance of and urgency for these simple procedures with hearing impaired children.

If an unexpected deterioration in the hearing occurs with no obvious simple cause, an urgent consultation with the ENT doctor is justified. Treatment may be appropriate, as perhaps may referral to an alternative centre specializing in these problems. It is important, as in all dealings with the parents, that those involved are honest about any changes in the hearing. Parents need to understand that it may not be known with complete certainty just how the hearing will behave over time, and they must realize that degeneration is not uncommon. Parents need to be aware that hearing aid retuning and alternative hearing aids are available to keep the hearing performance as good as possible. They should also be told that if the hearing were ever to become very poor, and hearing aid benefit became minimal, support to gain access to full information about all the alternative options for the future will be given. Parents may wish to pursue a cochlear implant referral in order to understand this possibility, or they may wish to learn about alternative communication strategies.

Conclusion

Despite the way in which we use the terms 'mild' and 'moderate' in our everyday conversations to mean something that is not of great significance, a mild or moderate hearing loss in children is a significant problem. Real difficulties, ranging through speech and language disruption, difficult behaviour and educational disadvantage, can greatly damage the quality of life of the child and the child's family. These effects have in the past sometimes been underrated. We now have the knowledge to avoid the damaging consequences of this problem if appropriate priority is given to the issues of early diagnosis and treatment.

References

Candlish P (1996) Not Deaf Enough: Raising a Child Who Is Hard of Hearing with Hugs, Humour and Imagination. Washington, DC: AG Bell Association for the Deaf.

Davies A, Bamford J, Wilson I, Ramkalawan T (1997) A critical review of the role of neonatal hearing screening in the detection of congenital hearing impairment. Health Technology Assessment 1(10).

Moore B (1995) Perceptual Consequences of Cochlear Damage. Oxford: Oxford Science Publications.

Chapter 5
Communication options

WENDY LYNAS

Deafness from birth imposes a severe threat to the development of language and communication. The most difficult decision confronting the parents of a recently diagnosed deaf child is the choice of communication approach; this is because 'communication' is crucial for so much else in life. The deaf child has the normal human capacity to develop language in all its complexity but can be prevented from realizing this potential for language by not having access to the speech of others. Language, which is acquired without much conscious effort by a child with normal hearing, can become an elusive goal for the young deaf child. Because of this, everyone agrees that the primary aim for deaf children is to 'unlock' the barrier to language and communication that deafness represents. There is, however, considerable disagreement on how to unlock that barrier.

There are, broadly speaking, three communication approaches currently in use in the UK: auditory-oral, total communication and bilingual. Those who advocate an auditory-oral approach argue that speech is accessible to the deaf child and that language and fluent communication can be acquired through the spoken word. Those who favour total communication (TC) claim that significant numbers of deaf children must have the support of signs if they are to communicate and acquire verbal language. Bilingualists consider it wrong that deaf children should have to struggle to acquire spoken language through the medium of a deficient hearing ability and believe that the entirely visual language of sign, which they claim is the natural language of the Deaf', should be made available to them as their first language.

These three approaches differ significantly in what they entail and in their overall objectives. Each of the different approaches requires a commitment of time and resources. To work effectively, each requires that it is begun early in the deaf child's life. The difficulty for parents is that they are forced to confront this choice concerning communication option early in the intervention process, at a time when they are feeling emotionally vulnerable and when they are unlikely to appreciate the full implications of their choice, implications that affect their role as parents and that will have a significant impact on the life-long future of their deaf child. The choice is made all the more difficult because of the complex moral and practical arguments for and against each of the three approaches.

The problem of choice is made even more difficult because of the disagreements, within the UK, between professionals and deaf people themselves about communication methods. This disagreement makes getting a dispassionate, non-biased judgement about the best method for a particular child very difficult for parents. In the circumstances, 'doing the best thing' for a deaf child entails getting to know as much as possible about the nature and implications of the available communication approaches. Parents need to be as well informed as possible if they are to take decisions on behalf of their own deaf child. Professionals, 'experts', will offer advice, but leaving the decision entirely to the 'experts' is not advisable: parents will feel undermined as parents if they do not play a major role in the decision-making. Parents need, as far as possible, to arm themselves against biased opinion and partisan advice.

The aim of this chapter is to offer information in as clear and impartial a way as possible in order to help parents and those who advise them to sort out the claims made on behalf of each of the three major communication options. Each of the three approaches – auditory-oral, total communication and bilingual – will in turn be described and examined to reveal the arguments used to support that particular method, its practical implications and the most recent available evidence concerning the educational outcome of the approach. The choice of options that are likely to be available in any particular child's local area will also be considered.

There are no absolutely clear solutions to the problem of giving deaf children communication and language or of providing them with educational opportunities equal to those of similar children with normal hearing. Nor are there any certain ways of knowing how young deaf children, as future adults, will want to live their lives. Yet, inevitably, a choice

---

*'Deaf' with an upper case D is now a widely accepted way of denoting cultural deafness and describes deaf people who elect to identify with the Deaf Community, who choose most of their significant social contact within a Deaf group and who communicate through sign language. The Deaf Community perceives itself to be a cultural and linguistic minority rather than a disabled group; for insight into the 'Deaf World', readers may like to read 'A Journey into the Deaf-World' by Lane et al. (1996). The term 'deaf' with a lower case d is broader and can refer to anyone with a significant hearing loss. For the purpose of this chapter, 'deaf' is not closely defined but refers, broadly speaking, to children or adults with hearing losses in the severe/profound category, i.e. of 70 dB or more.

of communication approach has to be made, and it is present-day adults who must make the decisions on behalf of deaf children. Because they are such fateful decisions, it is the duty of all concerned to examine the best available evidence before making that choice.

Auditory-oral approach

What is involved in the auditory-oral approach?

The central goal of the auditory-oral approach is communication through speech. This means making maximum use of deaf children's residual hearing and providing them with a facilitating spoken language environment.

Use of residual hearing

Those advocating an auditory-oral approach emphasize that total deafness in children – 'deaf from birth' – is extremely rare and that the overwhelming majority of profoundly deaf children therefore have some residual hearing. Modern oralists believe that the residual hearing of even the deafest of children can be exploited by means of systems of amplification so that the auditory processing parts of the brain can be activated and language can develop. It is acknowledged by oralists that even the best-quality hearing aids cannot restore normal hearing, but oralists claim that the spoken message, appropriately amplified, can provide an accessible and intelligible version of the message received by people with normal hearing.

It is considered extremely important that, as soon as the diagnosis of deafness is made, the child is fitted with appropriate hearing aids. Furthermore, it is extremely important that the hearing aids are kept in good working order and correctly worn. Parents should expect to receive immediate and regular support in the management of hearing aids from the local audiology clinic and the peripatetic service of teachers of the deaf.

Oralists claim that the minority of deaf children who have very little residual hearing or even no measurable hearing at all can, thanks to the development of cochlear implants, be enabled to perceive patterns of speech well enough to develop spoken language. Cochlear implantation requires surgery, but there is now in Britain a considerable amount of experience of performing this operation successfully on young children, as we will see in Chapter 6, and there are cochlear implant centres in most areas of the country.

Once the young infant's hearing is enhanced to the maximum, then, so oralists claim, the deaf child can start to perceive the speech of others so that spoken language development can begin.

Facilitating spoken language acquisition

The provision of good-quality language experience is a key aspect of the auditory-oral approach. All children need language experience if they are to acquire language, and deaf children need adequate and appropriate language input if they are to perceive what they hear as symbols of communication. It is very important that the spoken language surrounding the deaf child is relevant to his needs and interests. The language offered should be related to the child's focus of attention at any particular moment. If this is achieved, the deaf child will start to perceive the auditory signals as communication symbols. This, oralists acknowledge, is not as easy as it sounds. Talking to a child who does not readily respond to spoken communication is hard work. It is only too easy to become disheartened and not say very much. It is also easy to talk 'over the head' of the child or be overdirective, paying insufficient attention to what the child might be thinking or wanting to communicate (Gregory et al., 1979; Wood et al., 1986). Creating situations that require communicative exchange is part of the skill required by an adult in facilitating language acquisition. Parents can expect to receive support from the health and educational services in developing their communication skills with their young deaf child (Deaf Education through Listening and Talking, 1997).

Once adults develop a sensitivity to the deaf child's interests and communication needs, satisfying interaction can occur (Clark, 1989). The more the adult offers communication that is relevant to the deaf child's interests, the more, so it is claimed, the child will attend to speech and the more responsive and interactive he will become. Communicating with the deaf child gets progressively easier for the adult. The more deaf children develop their own capacity to listen, the more feedback they get from their own vocalizations, and this in itself encourages further vocalization. As the speech sounds received by the child come to be perceived as symbols of language and a means of communication, so the process of language acquisition gets under way.

Rationale of the auditory-oral approach

The moral case

The ideological position behind the auditory-oral approach is that verbal communication, particularly spoken communication, is the predominant medium of social exchange. Without the ability to speak and understand the speech of others, the individual's links with wider society are severely restricted.

Proponents of this approach agree that the deaf individual who knows sign language has a language, but they say this will permit communication only with other sign language users, who will, generally speaking, be deaf themselves. Deaf people do not live in exclusively Deaf neighbourhoods, nor are they employed in exclusively Deaf workplaces. Deaf adults are surrounded for most of the time by normally hearing people, and the demands of everyday life necessitate a considerable amount of exchange with people who speak and do not sign. If the life opportunities and objectives of the deaf person are to be as wide as those of other people, then, oralists argue, the deaf person needs to be able to interact with reasonable ease and confidence in spoken language.

The practical argument

The moral argument for the auditory-oral approach breaks down, of course, if the goal of speech for the deaf individual is found to be unachievable or achievable only by a minority of deaf children and young people. It is, however, claimed by those advocating an auditory-oral approach that it *is* possible to break through the barrier of deafness and that understanding and producing speech *is* a realistic goal for the overwhelming majority of even the deafest of children (Deaf Education through Listening and Talking, 1997). Moreover, if deaf children can communicate through spoken language, the foundation for literacy, and hence for educational development, is laid.

An evaluation of the auditory-oral approach

Advances in audiology and technology

So what support is there for the auditory-oral claim that deaf children can be enabled to talk and understand the speech of others? There have certainly been developments in technology and audiology over the past 10 or so years which mean that if we do want to harness the hearing of the deaf child for the development of spoken language, we are in a better position than ever to do so. Advances in measurement techniques and hearing aid technology mean that deaf children can be enabled to hear more effectively and from an earlier age.

The development of new techniques for measuring the hearing of babies during the first few days of life means that very early diagnosis is becoming more the norm in the UK for children with substantial and permanent hearing loss (Bamford and McSporran, 1993; Mauk and White, 1995).

Hearing aid technology has developed over the past 10 years: it has become possible to fit powerful hearing aids in the ears of very tiny babies (Hostler, 1987); hearing aids have become more powerful over a wider range of frequencies (Smith, 1997); hearing aids have become personalized and programmable (Smith, 1997); radio hearing aids (FM systems) have become more available and easier to use (Tucker and Powell, 1991); earmoulds give few problems of auditory feedback (Nolan and Tucker, 1988); and cochlear implants have become an increasingly important option for children with severe and profound hearing losses (see Chapter 6).

Developments in audiology and technology are believed by oralists to be crucial in enabling the deaf child to hear well enough to develop a valid representation of spoken language in the auditory processing parts of his brain. The auditory-oral approach depends also on the provision of appropriate language input in order for the language acquisition parts of the brain to be activated. Those advocating an auditory-oral approach believe that advances in our knowledge of verbal language acquisition have improved the prospects of success for the approach.

Advances in providing good language experience

Advances in the discipline of psycholinguistics mean that we now have much better knowledge of how language 'works' and how it is acquired. It is now known that language is 'caught' through the experience of language used in everyday contexts rather than 'taught' by instruction. The natural language used in the home can offer the young deaf child just the kind of language experience needed to facilitate the acquisition of spoken language. Oralists emphasize that all families in the UK should have access to a teacher, therapist and/or clinician who is trained to support spoken language interaction between parent and child (see Chapter 8).

The majority of severely and profoundly deaf children are now educated in mainstream schools, especially at the primary stage. Deaf children in the mainstream can benefit from the experience of language used by those who naturally communicate through talk: they are challenged not only to speak intelligibly, but also to make best use of their residual hearing in communicating with others (Harrison, 1993).

The outcomes of an auditory-oral approach

Modern oralists believe that the prospects of 'oral success' for the deaf child continue to improve year by year. Gone are the days, it is claimed, when the majority of deaf children left school with 'unintelligible' or 'very hard to understand' speech and reading ages of less than 9 years. This was the situation in the mid-1970s, according to a much-cited study by Conrad (1979), but it is now no longer the case. Conrad's study, which involved all deaf school-leavers in England and Wales, revealed that the majority of severely and profoundly deaf young people were leaving school without a command of the structures and vocabulary of the English language.

The oralism of the 1970s and before has rightly been criticized for its failure to offer fluent spoken communication and literacy to all but a minority of severely and profoundly deaf individuals. However, oralists claim that this criticism is no longer valid for more recently educated deaf children. So, can a judgement now be made about whether the potential benefits of recent advances in enhancing hearing and developing language are actually being realized?

Since some of the developments in knowledge, technology and services have existed for several years (Lynas, 1994), it should be the case that deaf children and young people who have been recently educated through an auditory-oral approach should be achieving fluent and intelligible oral communication and a mastery of verbal language and literacy. There is support from research within the past decade for the oralist conviction that there has been a genuine breakthrough in oral education, as outlined below.

A US study by Geers and Moog (1989) involved 100 hearing impaired young people from the USA and Canada, representing 50% of the orally educated young people aged 16–17 years in North America. All the subjects had a hearing loss greater than 85 dB HL; most (85%) were mainstreamed for all or most of the day. The results showed an average reading age of 13–14 years, only 15% having a reading age of around 8 years or less. Eighty-eight per cent demonstrated proficiency with spoken English from both a language and speech intelligibility point of view.

A UK study involved an analysis of the written language of 28 orally educated children in Leicestershire aged 5–17 years with hearing losses greater than 90 dB HL (Harrison et al., 1991). Twenty-two of the children produced written language that was judged to demonstrate a 'fluent and expressive use of complex language allowing easy extraction of meaning'. Clearly, 22 out of the 28 were achieving genuine literacy. Of the remaining six who were less competent writers, none was above the age of 11 years 5 months, so it is likely that some of these children were displaying immaturity in their writing and would in time improve.

The other UK study involved 82 orally educated young people aged 15–17 years with severe and profound hearing losses (Lewis, 1996). Overall, the hearing losses of the young people featuring in Lewis's sample were greater than those in Conrad's study, described above. Lewis used the same reading measures as Conrad (1979), so that direct comparisons could be made. The median reading age of Lewis's group was 13 years 4 months, compared with that of Conrad's sample, which was less than 9 years. Only 14.6% of Lewis's group had a reading age of 9 years or less. Lewis's median reading age is considerably above that of Conrad's sample: most of Lewis's sample were achieving genuine literacy, whereas most of Conrad's sample were not.

All three studies cited support the oralist argument that there has been progress with oral education since it is now the *majority* of deaf children and young people who are achieving mastery of verbal language rather than a minority achieving oral success, as was the case at the time of Conrad's study. Despite this, research evidence support for the use of an exclusively auditory-oral approach with all deaf children is still currently criticized by some people. It is important, therefore, to outline what are perceived to be the drawbacks of the pure oralist position.

Difficulty of putting the auditory-oral approach into practice

All three approaches examined in this chapter require commitment on the part of parents and professionals if they are to work to best effect, and the auditory-oral approach is no exception. In the early years, it is crucial that hearing aids are managed correctly, and this is no easy task. Taking care of these relatively small, fiddly technical devices that can easily go wrong or break requires time, skill and patience. Keeping the hearing aid in the ear of the deaf infant who rejects this 'foreign body' can be a problem.

For the deaf child, learning to appreciate that what at first might seem like faint muffled noises are actually symbols of communication, takes time. Developing an easy interaction between the parent and child can be a problem in the early stages.

Despite these potential and often very real difficulties, those in favour of the auditory-oral approach claim that, with skill and sensitivity, satisfying interaction can take place between the deaf child and other family members (Clark, 1989). The frustration caused by failures to communicate is not an inevitable part of the early life of the young deaf child. The auditory-oral approach alone requires parents and other family members to talk to the deaf child using their own language, and this goes some way towards enabling comfortable communication. Commitment is required, but no more than would be required by any of the other approaches. (Indeed, the amount and complexity of this form of intervention is arguably less than that required by either of the other two approaches.)

Language delay

Oralists acknowledge that, in the preschool years, profoundly deaf children do not learn to listen and acquire language immediately they are fitted with hearing aids: spoken language acquisition takes longer than when a child has normal hearing.

Children with normal hearing, on reaching school age, typically have a sizeable vocabulary and mastery of the structures or grammar of their native language. Schools do not generally see it as part of their role to contribute to the basic process of language acquisition. The deaf child, with linguistic structures still to acquire and a relatively small vocabulary, can be seen to be at a disadvantage because he is linguistically less well equipped to receive the education that is offered.

The response of oralists to the problem of language delay for deaf children in the early years is that the delay does not seem to prevent their eventually mastering the structures of verbal language. This is confirmed by research elsewhere that if there is a 'critical period' for language acquisition, it is not the first 5 years of life (Bishop and Mogford, 1993). Clearly, at school age, the deaf child needs continuing support with the acquisition of the grammar and vocabulary of language, and it is essential that teachers and parents maintain their efforts at fostering language learning both at home and at school. The social and learning environment of the infant school, with its many opportunities for social interaction with other children and adults, will, it is argued, significantly promote the language development of the deaf child.

The problem of everyday communication

Even if we are satisfied that the deaf child is making appropriate progress with spoken language development and literacy, there is still the problem, particularly at a mainstream school, of having to communicate throughout the day in spoken language. The mainstreamed deaf child or young person is surrounded by competent hearer-speakers and is likely to be reminded frequently of his hearing disability through the frustrations of failures to grasp all that is being said and through his inability to participate fully in the cut-and-thrust of informal school life.

The problem of access to the curriculum

It can be argued that to receive an education exclusively through speech means a constant struggle for the deaf pupil. The deaf child is always at a disadvantage relative to hearing children in receiving information via the spoken word: the deaf child must concentrate harder with both eyes and ears to keep abreast of lesson material (Lynas, 1986).

Those in favour of an oral communication approach acknowledge that it is undoubtedly difficult to be deaf in a hearing society but argue that an oral education offers the best preparation for participation in the hearing world. Acquiring an education through oral means is not easy, but, so far, the oral approach seems to offer the widest educational opportunities in terms of academic achievement. Testimony from a profoundly deaf young person, reporting on her success in higher education, offers support for an oral education:

Indeed, it is true that if I had not been educated orally, I would not be where I am now. This is sad but a fact of life which perhaps British Sign Language supporters do not recognise ... We must be realistic as deaf people do form a minority in society and thus we cannot expect all hearing people to learn Sign Language for the benefit of a few deaf people whom they may never encounter anyway. (Briggs, 1991, p. 109)

Those deaf children and young people who are educated in mainstream schools, particularly if they are individually integrated into their local school, need special support: they must not be left to flounder academically or socially, and they need to retain a healthy self-confidence. A range of support is available from the visiting teacher of the deaf service, and fortunately a more 'inclusive' climate is developing in many schools. Where there is an 'inclusive' ethos, all pupils, regardless of difference or disability, are welcome, and it is considered the role of the school to adapt itself in order to educate *all* children (Ainscow, 1995).

Persistence of oral 'failure'

A dilemma for oralists concerns whether or not all deaf children can achieve acceptable levels of language and communication through an auditory-oral approach. Some children who are deaf have very little residual hearing; a significant number of deaf children have additional problems such as physical or learning difficulties (Schildroth and Hotto, 1991); some deaf children, despite good amplification and good language input, seem to find using their hearing for the development of intelligible spoken language extremely difficult. For example, there were a minority of the sample involved in the studies of Geers and Moog (1989) and Lewis (1996), cited above, who did not achieve proficiency in spoken language and did not achieve literacy. Some writers think that there are differences in children's psycho-perceptual abilities and that when a child is very deaf, this feature can have an overwhelming influence on the ability of some children to make use of their residual hearing (Ling, 1976; Bamford and Saunders, 1991).

If there are 'within-child' features that, regardless of the auditory and linguistic environment, will limit the development of oral communicative competence, it would be useful to be able to diagnose these features at an early stage in the child's life in order to allow alternative communication options to be used effectively. However, it does not seem as if any reliable diagnostic technique exists. Ross (in Luterman, 1991) has observed that:

some 'deaf children' are visual learners who want and can use the unambiguous signal provided by a sign system, whilst others are

capable of using their residual hearing very well ... what is needed
is a period of experimental teaching to find out which is the best
method ... audiograms can be poor predictors of success in a
particular programme: children with very severe losses do quite
well aurally, while other children with more pure tone hearing
don't do nearly as well.

On the issue of when to take the decision that oralism is 'failing' a
deaf child, there is no agreement. Oralists might accept the principle
that there is no one method suitable for all children but would argue,
irrespective of this, that all children, however deaf, should be given the
chance to develop oral language through a natural auditory approach
since we do not know in the early stages how well a child can hear or
discriminate speech. If we do not offer an auditory-oral approach, we
may lose for ever the chance to enable the child to learn to listen and
perceive speech. Developments in cochlear implantation offer fresh
support to oralists for the idea that all deaf children can be enabled to
hear and discriminate speech.

Lack of respect for Deaf identity

An issue considered particularly serious by many critics of oralism is that
the basis underlying an oral education, particularly an oral education in
the mainstream, is *morally* wrong. An oral education, it is alleged,
implies that the deaf child should assimilate into the hearing world and
conform as far as possible to the norms of hearing society. This 'denies
deafness' and implies an attempt to make a deaf child be what he can
never be: a hearing person (Ladd, 1988). Encouraging the deaf child to
take on the social identity of a hearing person is to deny the child access
to his 'true' identity, which is that of a Deaf person.

Oralists respond to this criticism by agreeing that deafness *does*
impose certain limitations in a hearing society. Oralists also acknowledge that encouraging deaf children to associate with hearing children
and adults is likely to foster identification with those who can hear, but
they do not agree that this is a bad thing: to become accustomed to
being deaf in a hearing world from an early age is believed by oralists to
be beneficial. Oralists, supportive of mainstream education for deaf children, reject the accusation that an ordinary school education implies a
'denial' of deafness and that it forces on the deaf an unnatural social
experience. On the contrary, an education in the mainstream, so the
oralist argument goes, allows the mutual acceptance of deaf and hearing
individuals and a shared respect for differences. Both deaf and hearing
children have the opportunity to learn that we are all different in some
respects and that we all have weaknesses and strengths. Furthermore,
whilst growing up in the midst of hearing people does not, it is true,

promote a sense of belonging to the Deaf community or of having a special 'Deaf' identity, there are plenty of opportunities for the deaf individual to become part of the 'Deaf World' as they grow up if they want to do so. No-one is stopping the deaf child/young person from learning sign language or joining the local Deaf club if he so wishes. The use of an auditory-oral approach allows the deaf individual, so advocates argue, participation in the wider society and all the very many cultural and interest groups that exist within a society such as Britain, as well as permitting identification with the Deaf group if that is the individual's wish.

We can see that the pure auditory-oral approach is not without its problems, but advocates would argue that it is the best option 'on balance'. Those who favour a TC approach disagree. They argue that some deaf children need the visual medium of sign in order to communicate; that the use of sign can eliminate or reduce the delay in language acquisition that is typically a feature of a pure auditory-oral approach; and that signs can be used to support the development of spoken language and literacy. The claims of the TC approach will be presented next.

Total communication

What is involved in a TC approach?

TC involves the use of all methods of communication – sign, gesture, finger-spelling, speech, hearing, lip movements and facial expression. Signs, finger-spelling and so on do not *replace* speech and the use of hearing; the idea is that visual communication will *support* audition and speech. Speech and signs, sight and hearing, work together in a TC approach.

The signs used in a TC approach are taken from the sign languages used by members of the Deaf Community in a particular country. So, for example, in the UK, the signs are drawn from British Sign Language (BSL), in the USA from American Sign Language (ASL). The sign system in a TC approach is not the same as the natural sign languages that have been evolved over the years by deaf people and which have a very different structure from the structure of English or any verbal language. BSL is not, therefore, a manual-visual form of English and is not suitable for use simultaneously with speech. The signing used in a TC or signs-and-speech approach in the UK is a contrived system of 'content' signs drawn from BSL that are presented in English word order with additional invented signs to represent English syntactic features, for example verb inflections such as 'ing' and 'ed', and function words such 'the', 'as' and 'of'. Where there is no BSL sign corresponding to a word in English, finger-spelling is used to supplement signs.

Advocates of TC argue that signs should be used in the home from early infancy: the deaf infant, like any other, uses his eyes to scan the environment, to notice objects and events. If caregivers can offer signs and gestures in response to the infant's visual attention, they not only develop satisfying interaction and communication, but also provide readily accessible linguistic symbols. TC means *total* communication, and that means that the deaf child's residual hearing should be exploited with the best-quality amplification. Hearing aids are, in principle, as important in a TC approach as in an auditory-oral one. Deaf children should be encouraged to listen as well as look. It is, of course, necessary for parents to learn to sign, and in the UK there are many classes where some form of sign is taught. The LEA hearing impaired service should have information about local facilities for learning sign, and some will offer sign classes themselves. It is believed that the reward of being able to communicate easily with their deaf child, without stress or frustration, will provide ample reward for parents for taking the trouble to learn sign.

Many supporters of TC believe that, far from detracting from the development of spoken language, the early use of signs *facilitates communication*, so that speech can emerge when the child is ready. The pressure to use and receive speech, and only speech, is removed: by being able to use sign and gesture in the early years, the deaf child gains confidence in communication and is better able to cope with the difficult task of receiving and producing speech.

TC is a flexible approach and can be adapted to the needs of individual children, some children needing to rely on the signed component more than others. Parents, teachers and others who use a TC approach can adjust their speech and signing to suit the different needs of different children at different stages of their development.

TC used in schools by teachers of the deaf, support-assistants or interpreters will ensure, so advocates of TC claim, a continued development of language and full access to the curriculum. Presenters of signs in accompaniment to speech must, of course, be competent signers and have a sufficiently rich vocabulary to offer an enriched language input. They should, through TC, be able to support full access to the ideas and information taught in schools.

As originally conceived (Denton, 1976), TC used in a formal educational context required the simultaneous use of speech and a signed version of every element of the spoken message. Thus, a teacher of the deaf, with a group of deaf children, would be expected to speak and sign simultaneously the content of the curriculum using full linguistic forms. However, because of the intrinsic difficulty of combining speech uttered at a normal rate with a signed version of that speech (Baker, 1978; Wood and Wood, 1992), a more generally accepted interpretation of TC means using signs to *support* the spoken message. The aim of using signs in support of speech is to clarify the spoken message, lessen ambiguity and emphasize new or key words rather than provide a complete manual-visual language. The deaf school or college pupil who is offered signs in support of speech will not, so it is argued, have to struggle to follow the curriculum, as is the case with a pure auditory-oral approach. Where deaf children are being educated in mainstream schools, support teachers or support assistants can, through the use of signs offered at appropriate times during the lesson, explain difficult concepts and vocabulary presented by the class teacher.

Signs can also be used to teach grammatical forms and help develop literacy. A problem for the deaf child acquiring language is that syntactic elements – words such as 'a', 'the' and 'of', and word endings such as 'ed' and 's', are, in connected speech, the least audible sounds. Grammatical elements can be presented to the deaf child in a visual form and thereby give them 'total' linguistic information, in contrast to speech alone, which gives only 'partial' linguistic information. The development of literacy can be helped by the use of signs to decode and encode the written word.

Rationale for a TC approach

TC involves the use of sign as well as speech in order to develop the language and communication of deaf children. By making use of the visual medium of sign, one is making use of the sense of vision to supplement and support the deaf child's faulty hearing. This will, it is believed, inevitably improve communication and linguistic understanding. A TC approach, it is claimed, will get 'the best of all worlds' from a communication point of view.

It is easy to see the appeal of TC: signs are 100% accessible to the deaf child, yet speech is always heard imperfectly. When TC was introduced in the UK in the late 1970s, advocates held that the pure oral approach was directly responsible for the low educational and linguistic standards typically achieved by deaf young people and that there was a clear-cut case for the use of sign in the education of deaf children. Thus, despite technological advances in amplification, TC supporters believe that some deaf children are simply too deaf to perceive spoken language through the auditory channel alone. The TC approach, on the other hand, offers a deaf child easy communication through sign and, it is claimed, access to the symbols of verbal language. Inevitably, so it is argued, the educational standards of deaf children will be raised with the adoption of the TC principle.

An evaluation of the TC approach

Since we have had many years of experience of TC practice, both in the USA and the UK, we ought to be in a position to judge the effectiveness of the approach. One problem with evaluating TC, however, is that 'total communication', to an extent, means 'all things to all people' and practices in the name of TC are very varied.

Use of signs and gesture at the early stages of communication development

Some research in the UK indicates that gesture and sign may have a constructive role to play in the deaf child's progression to speech but that this progression is the same for all children, deaf or hearing (Robinshaw, 1992).

Robinshaw examined the transition from non-communicative behaviour to language production in five deaf and five matched hearing infants. For all the infants, deaf and hearing, the use of communicative gesture formed an important step from presymbolic to symbolic language. The deaf infants' use of gesture as a primary means of communication continued over a longer period compared with the hearing infants, but the pattern of development was the same for both groups. The deaf children's use of gesture declined as their auditory perception improved and their attempts at speech became more intelligible to caregivers. Robinshaw suggests, however, that once the deaf child begins to perceive and discriminate auditorily, the continued use of sign and gesture will have a detrimental effect on the development of auditory discrimination and vocal/verbal development.

Combining signs and speech to advance verbal language development

There is accumulating evidence that seems to confirm Robinshaw's (1992) suggestion that using a combination of speech and signs to promote language acquisition beyond the early stages is not producing the hoped-for results in relation to the overall language and educational achievements of deaf children and young people. Let us look at these findings.

Whilst early language and communication seem to be helped, or at least not hindered, by the use of sign, a US study by Bornstein and Saulnier (1981) indicated that the continued use of sign slows down verbal language development.

Profoundly deaf children educated consistently with some form of signed English and speech have been shown to be inferior in terms of speech and language compared with profoundly deaf children educated consistently with an auditory-oral approach (Geers et al., 1984; Markides, 1988).

Large-scale surveys of the attainments of deaf children and young people in the USA indicate that TC-educated young people are leaving school with standards of literacy and speech achievements that are no higher than those of deaf young people leaving school in the 1960s and 70s, that is, before the introduction of TC (Schildroth and Hotto, 1991).

This finding from the USA, which involves very large numbers of deaf children, is perhaps the greatest condemnation of all of TC. If the overwhelming majority of TC-educated young people are leaving school with reading ages of between 8 and 9 years and with very poor speech, TC, at least as it has been practised, has failed in its own terms: it has been unsuccessful in delivering verbal language to deaf children.

Problems with the TC approach

It is significant that, during the 1980s, corresponding with the reports of low attainments of TC-educated children, more and more research has emerged revealing problems with both the principles and practice of TC.

A spoken language such as English takes about twice as long to articulate in a signed form as it does in the spoken form. Hence, it is intrinsically impossible to speak English at a normal rate and sign at the same time. Transcripts of speech-and-signs indicate that there are distortions of both the spoken and the signed components. Typically, speech is slowed down and signs are omitted (Baker, 1978). The most probable omissions of signs are those denoting the grammatical features of English (Marmor and Pettito, 1979; Wood and Wood, 1992). So, whilst TC is supposed to offer 'total' linguistic information, it seems that there are intrinsic reasons why it cannot.

Many teachers presenting signs and speech find it difficult in practice to convey the meaning of what they say in signed form (Kluwin, 1981). This seems to have the effect of restricting the language input to deaf pupils (Huntington and Watton, 1984). Teachers have been observed to avoid 'difficult' vocabulary and grammatical structures in both the signed and the spoken form (Newton, 1985; Lai and Lynas, 1991), thereby doing the very opposite of what is often claimed for the TC approach – ensuring vocabulary enrichment and development of language structures.

Children who are educated through a combination of speech and some signed version of that speech have been observed to use neither in their everyday communication (Gee and Goodhart, 1988). Outside the classroom, when deaf children and young people are communicating 'for real', they are observed to 'nativize' their signing so that it becomes more like the natural sign languages used within the Deaf Community.

There is, then, some qualified support for the use of TC. Gestures and signs may provide an effective route into verbal language at the early stages of communication, which may be particularly important for some children who have additional disabilities or learning difficulties. However, many people who believed that a combination of speech and signs would provide a solution to the problem of giving language to deaf children are now fiercely critical of TC (e.g. Hansen, 1990; Lane et al., 1996).

TC is clearly more difficult to put into practice than was at first realized. Some of the difficulties almost certainly lie in the deficiencies of the signing ability of many teachers and parents. Those who are attempting to support language and communication for deaf children through sign ought to be competent signers, but frequently they are not: parents do not always have the time or resources to devote to learning a 'new' language (Bornstein et al., 1980). Teachers who offer restricted linguistic input when using TC do so in part because of their lack of knowledge and fluency in sign (Kluwin, 1981; Newton 1985). However, as we have seen, some of the difficulties are intrinsic to simultaneous communication.

Overall, TC is having a hard time at present, and no-one seems particularly interested in 'perfecting' the practice of combining speech with signed speech (Mahshie, 1995). Those who support the auditory-oral approach believe that they are vindicated and are correct in their beliefs that signs do not, generally speaking, contribute to the deaf child's acquisition of verbal language. But many who condemn TC believe very strongly that signs *should* be used to develop language and communication in deaf children but *not* in combination with speech (Mahshie, 1995; Baker, 1997). Bilingualists believe that sign language should be the first and primary language of deaf children, and they now form a strong lobby in the communication debate.

Bilingual approach

Bilingualism has attracted much recent attention and can be seen as a reaction against both the auditory-oral and TC approaches. The auditory-oral approach, it is claimed, fails to meet the language and communication needs of children who are born deaf and imposes on them a system of communication in which they are always at a disadvantage. TC, as it has been practised, not only fails to bring verbal language to deaf children, but also offers only an artificially contrived form of sign: a manual-visual form of English does not constitute a 'proper' language.

A 'real' language that can meet the linguistic and communication needs of deaf children does exist, say bilingualists, and that is the sign language used by Deaf people within their own group. Natural sign languages, such as BSL, have been analysed by linguists and judged to be 'proper' languages, with the same capacity as any verbal language for the expression of ideas (Stokoe, 1960). Bilingualists believe that access to 'the natural language of the deaf' is the birthright of all deaf children. Bilingualists support the goal of verbal language, at least in the written form, but believe that verbal language will, for most deaf children, need to be taught as a second language. It is claimed that, once sign language is established, sign language itself can be used as a means of acquiring a second language such as English (Cummins and Swain, 1986).

What is involved in a bilingual approach?

Language acquisition

Bilingualists are insistent that deaf children should be offered sign language input as soon as their deafness is diagnosed (Mahshie, 1995; Baker, 1997). But how does the newly diagnosed deaf infant get access to sign language? The majority of children who are born with severe and profound hearing losses – around 90% in Britain – have hearing parents who are unlikely to know sign language. This is, of course, a problem if BSL is to be offered as a first language.

This problem is not treated lightly by bilingualists, and they acknowledge that the parents of deaf children need considerable support, information and guidance to help them and their children to become bilingual (Mahshie, 1995). Parents, and indeed other members of the family, need to be given the opportunity to attend BSL classes in their local area, to attend weekend courses and to attend local Deaf Clubs. Appropriately placed centres need to be established where deaf toddlers and infants can attend, preferably with their parents, and where they will be 'immersed' in sign. The centres would comprise older deaf children, deaf adults, signing teachers and signing parents (Johnson et al., 1989; Mahshie, 1995). Signing can be brought into the home by those who can sign fluently: Deaf adults can spend time interacting in sign with the young deaf child and can offer support to parents in learning sign language.

It is claimed that, when the deaf child starts to communicate in sign, the parents are likely to form a positive view of their deaf child's abilities and cease to regard him as a handicapped child (Bouvet, 1990). This in itself will provide parents with the motivation to develop their own sign language skills.

BSL as the medium of education

The bilingualist goal is for the deaf child, on reaching 5 years of age, to be at the same level of language in sign as the hearing child is in speech. Assuming that this goal has been realized, it is necessary to offer deaf children the school curriculum in sign. Whether in a special or a mainstream school, the deaf child needs a generous supply of trained signing teachers, including deaf teachers, signing interpreters and signing classroom assistants. With such provision, the deaf child will have the same opportunity as the hearing child to acquire knowledge and 'achieve' academically. It is considered important that the deaf child should have access to a variety of sign users, both children and adults, during the course of the day in order to sustain language growth. In Scandinavian countries, where there is over 15 years' experience of offering a bilingual approach to deaf children, this is taken to mean that deaf children should be educated in special schools for the deaf (Bergman and Wallin, 1994). However, given that there is a strong tradition in the UK of educating deaf children in the mainstream, UK bilingualists do not necessarily believe that a special school is essential (Pickersgill, 1997). However, for deaf children to get sufficient input of sign language with maximum use being made of the scarce resources of Deaf adults, inter-preters and signing teachers, it is considered important that they are grouped together in a unit or resource centre within a mainstream school (British Deaf Association, 1996). This also gives the deaf child access to a Deaf peer group (Pickersgill, 1997).

Developing literacy

With the bilingual approach, the goal of literacy in English has to be achieved by teaching the deaf child English as a second language. Bilin-gualists acknowledge that making the transition between BSL and written English, which has a completely different structure from that of any sign language, is not easy to achieve (Pickersgill, 1997). However, there are some ideas about how to bridge the gap between sign language and the majority verbal language (Mahshie, 1995; Strong, 1995; Pickersgill, 1997).

Pickersgill (1997) suggests that manually coded English can play a role in translating BSL into English. Furthermore, it is believed that chil-dren of school age are capable of analysing the structure of their own language use and are thus in a position to understand the structure of another language. The principle of developing an understanding of the structure of one's first language in order to facilitate the learning of another is well accepted in second language teaching (Cummins and Swain, 1986; Ahlgren, 1994; Strong, 1995).

The principles of 'exposure' and 'comprehensible input' (Krashen, 1982) are considered important in second language learning generally and are believed to be important in teaching English as a second language to deaf children. Deaf children need to be encouraged to pay attention to the 'words' in their environment, for example on cereal packets, in shop windows and in advertisements, magazines, newspa-pers, books, etc. Videos with captions and books with pictures can be useful ways of linking something that is comprehensible visually with the written word. Children can be told stories in sign and, when familiar with the content of a story, be presented with written text. Words can be 'read' and 'discussed' using sign language. In this way, written English will be introduced in the comprehensible context of sign language, and deaf children will be enabled to come to understand text in their own time in a relaxed and non-pressured way.

The role of speech in a bilingual approach

There seem to be differences of opinion, or at least emphasis, amongst bilingualists concerning the development of speech in deaf children. The following appear to reflect what currently seem to be the different viewpoints.

First, since speech is an unattainable goal for deaf children, or at best one that can only be obtained with great difficulty, time should not be 'wasted' in trying to achieve the 'virtually impossible'. Since sign language and written language serve the linguistic, educational and communication needs of the deaf individual, speech need not be considered an essential goal (Johnson et al., 1989).

Second, all deaf children, since they live in a hearing-speaking world, will be exposed in their everyday lives to a considerable amount of speech. If the deaf child has some natural ability to acquire speech, he will use speech as a means of communication in some contexts (Axelsson, 1994).

Third, the development of spoken English should not be left to chance: deaf children should be given maximum opportunities to use their residual hearing and should therefore be given the best possible amplification and access to situations where spoken language is used as a means of communication (Jansma et al., 1997). 'Live' English as well as written English should be a target language (Pickersgill, 1997). Most deaf children will move in both the hearing-speaking worlds and the Deaf-signing worlds. It is considered to be a very important principle that the two forms of communication should be separated: sign language should be used in contexts where sign is the primary means of communication and should come to be associated in the deaf child's mind with particular people; spoken language should be associated with speaking people (Jansma et al., 1997). Deaf children, like other bilingual children in the world, will become sociolinguistically competent (Volterra and Taeschner, 1978) and appreciate when sign is required and when it is appropriate to use oral communication.

Rationale for the bilingual approach

The rationale for a bilingual approach has a strong ideological component. A bilingual approach for deaf children is not just an alternative method, but also represents a new way of thinking about deaf individuals (Pickersgill, 1997). Bilingualism, it is argued, is a philosophy that honours the right of deaf children to their own language. Within the bilingual approach, sign is *not* a mere prop to support speech, nor, it is emphasized, is it a last resort for children who 'fail' with other methods. Deaf children who are offered sign language as their first language are, so bilingualists claim, free from disability. With sign language, children can develop a distinct Deaf identity of which they can be proud (Lane et al., 1996). The bilingual model, unlike the auditory-oral model or TC, is not based on a 'deficit' view of the deaf child. Deaf children are different rather than deficient, but in the past, so the argument goes, they have been dis-abled by educators who have sought to impose their hearing-speaking norms on deaf individuals. The deaf individual can never be equal in situations where speech is the medium of exchange. To insist that deaf children receive their education in a language that is not fully developed and difficult to access is a violation of their rights to receive an education in their own language.

With sign language, the deaf individual can communicate as effectively as anyone else. Sign language, it is claimed, is uniquely suited to the abilities of the deaf individual, and it is *only*, bilingualists emphasize, by offering sign language as a first language that the young deaf child can acquire language without delay. Age-appropriate language, bilingualists argue, is a fundamental right of the deaf child and an essential objective of the bilingual approach. When the deaf child reaches the same milestones of language acquisition in sign as the hearing child achieves with speech, and if they have access to the full curriculum delivered in sign, then, for the first time in the history of deaf education, Deaf children and young people will have genuine equality of opportunity in education. This point is emphasized by the BDA in their education policy statement:

> Deaf people have the right to a quality education throughout their lives, which accepts their linguistic, cultural and social identity, which builds positive self-esteem and which sets no limit to their learning. (British Deaf Association, 1996)

Bilingualists argue that the use of sign language as a first language and medium of education is what deaf people themselves want. What the adult Deaf Community in Britain demand is the right of future generations of deaf individuals to their 'natural' language as a primary means of communication (British Deaf Association, 1996). Deaf people are claiming the right to be stake-holders in the education of deaf children, with the view that deaf education should no longer be the exclusive preserve of teachers of the deaf (British Deaf Association, 1996).

Bilingualists argue that, when BSL becomes the British deaf child's first language, sign language can be used to teach English as a second language. In this way, the deaf child has access to verbal language and literacy. There is nothing unusual about this principle: over half of the world's population are bilingual or multilingual and millions of children learn to read in a language that is not their mother tongue (Baker, 1997).

An evaluation of the bilingual approach

Bilingual education for deaf children in the UK is in its early days, but there has nonetheless been some critical appraisal of the principles of the approach (Lynas, 1994), much careful reflection on the practice (Strong, 1995; British Association of Teachers of the Deaf, 1997) and some outcome data from Sweden and Denmark (Mahshie, 1995).

Providing sufficient sign language input in the early years

Given that the majority of deaf children are born into a home environment where communication is through speaking, there is a serious practical problem in offering the deaf infant and young child sufficient sign language input in the crucial early years of language acquisition. Parents have to be willing to devote time and effort to learning sign, and it cannot be assumed that all parents will have the time or be prepared to make that effort. Even if parents are enthusiastic about learning sign language, they need considerable support from sign language classes, signing teachers and Deaf adults in order to acquire BSL sufficiently well to be able to communicate comfortably and fluently with their deaf child as BSL is harder to learn than a signed version of English. If parents do not sign much with their deaf child, and the deaf child acquires his knowledge of sign outside the home, this could undermine the bonds between the deaf child and his family: parents are likely to feel unconfident in communicating with their deaf child and even feel alienated from him. A recent longitudinal study in Bristol of deaf children educated bilingually indicates that, for their hearing parents, 'It is difficult to learn to sign. It is difficult to accept the otherness of one's child' (Ackerman et al., 1997).

In Sweden and Denmark, however, educators claim great success in encouraging hearing parents to learn the new language of sign (Mahshie, 1995). Parents in Denmark and Sweden receive extremely generously funded support from the state, as well as from parents' organizations and the Deaf Community, for learning sign language and for sharing in the education of their deaf children. It has been pointed out that both countries are affluent, with long histories of comprehensive state-funded health, education and welfare and 'excellent services for individuals with a variety of disabilities' (Mahshie, 1995).

The attainment of age-appropriate language

The promise of age-appropriate language by the age of 5 years is an appealing feature of the bilingual approach. The question is, can this promise be fulfilled? Does sign language acquisition follow the same timetable as the acquisition of spoken language?

Unfortunately, we do not have data, even from Scandinavia, on the language attainments of significant numbers of bilingually reared 5- or 6-year-old deaf children. There are reports of individual children developing sign symbols at the early stages of linguistic development in a similar way to that of hearing children acquiring vocal symbols (Gallaway and Woll, 1994). However, one British study, undertaken by Harris et al. (1989), throws some doubt on whether all deaf children exposed to sign language in the early years develop sign language as quickly as hearing children acquire spoken language, even when the parents are themselves deaf and use sign.

The investigation involved observations of four profoundly deaf children together with their profoundly deaf mothers. In all cases, the children's deafness had been diagnosed before the age of 3 months, and BSL was the main language of the home. The children were observed at intervals between the ages of 7 months and 2 years. The sign language development of the children was recorded, and, whilst there were variations, all the children were, for their age, considerably behind what is average in spoken language development for children with normal hearing (Harris et al., 1989).

There is clearly a need for more large-scale studies of the acquisition of sign language in young deaf children. A problem in conducting such studies, however, is that there are no agreed and accepted ways of assessing the development of vocabulary and grammar in natural sign language (Jansma et al., 1997). Whilst work is going on in this very important area (Jansma et al., 1997), there is at the moment no validated scale of norms for the acquisition of sign language by which to judge the level of sign language achieved by the individual deaf child. This means that monitoring linguistic progress in sign is problematic at the early stages of linguistic development and indeed throughout all stages of education.

Offering an education in sign language

That deaf children can get access to education in 'their own language', in the language of their everyday communication, is a further attractive feature of bilingualism. However, experience in Britain and elsewhere indicates that implementing the policy of delivering an education in sign language is extremely problematic (Baker, 1997; Jansma et al., 1997).

Baker (1997) has pointed out that the supply of teachers and interpreters who are fluent in sign language in Britain is limited. The majority of courses of training for teachers of the deaf in Britain do not offer sign language tuition as a central part of the training (Pickersgill, 1997). The supply of certificated sign language interpreters is increasing but is insufficient to meet the demands of a policy of bilingual education for all deaf children in the UK. If every deaf child were to receive the entire school curriculum delivered in sign language, there would be nowhere near enough appropriately skilled and qualified personnel to go round.

Are these 'practical problems to be overcome rather than problems of principle that are insurmountable' (Baker, 1997), or will the scale of the resource difficulty defeat the bilingual purpose? Bilingualists believe that involving many more Deaf adults in the education of deaf children, and offering a considerable amount of in-service training to teachers, will 'win through' in the end. It is acknowledged that there are major obstacles but that:

> we are approaching a threshold beyond which the momentum of the movement will carry it through; a time when bilingualism will be acknowledged as an imperative and when it will no longer rely on the efforts of the few but will be the way of life of the many. (Pickersgill, 1997)

Literacy achievements

Mahshie (1995) cites some evidence from Sweden and Denmark on the literacy outcomes of bilingually educated deaf pupils.

> Hansen (1990) examined the reading attainments of a group of 12-year-old pupils while they were in the process of being educated bilingually. She reported that 55% of them were able to 'read for meaning' and that a further 23% read at a 'transitional' stage. She compares these achievements with those in the past in Denmark when only 10–15% learnt to read for meaning by the time they left school.

> Salander and Svendenfors (1993), reporting from Sweden, evaluated the reading and writing abilities of nine 10th grade (16-year-old) pupils who had been bilingually educated from their preschool years. They had all learnt Swedish as a second language. Salander and Svendenfors found that, in reading, 3 were above average for their age, 5 average and 1 below average. In terms of writing, 3 were above average, 1 average and 5 below average.

> Heiling (1990) reported on tests of all 8th grade (14-year-old) pupils at Lund School for the Deaf in Sweden from 1985 to 1989 and concluded that 'subjects from the eighties were superior to their deaf age-mates from twenty years earlier in all tests measuring ability to understand and use written Swedish'.

Beyond the evidence cited above, however, there is little apart from anecdotal reports. Thus, we are looking at the literacy attainments of a very small deaf population. We really need evidence on the literacy outcomes of a larger group. Then we will be able to judge with more confidence whether or not learning verbal language through sign language *is* possible for the majority of deaf children. It may or may not be significant that reports of large-scale studies from Denmark and

Sweden are not available. Knoors (1997), reviewing a book based on a conference in Sweden in 1993 on 'Bilingualism in Deaf Education', notes an absence of contributions based on achievement data: 'Alas, there were virtually no data, and far too much rhetoric.'

It is gratifying that, in the UK, there is a planned survey of the educational achievements of all children with sensorineural hearing loss at different ages and stages of education, supported by the Royal National Institute for the Deaf (Tymms, 1997). Children with significant hearing loss in the UK are educated by a variety of means, and it is to be hoped that the proposed research will help unravel factors, for example communication approach, that are significant to the attainments of British deaf children.

The goal of speech

As we have seen, the goal and the role of speech in the bilingual deaf child's communication development is differently emphasized amongst those who support bilingualism. The view currently presented in the UK (British Association of Teachers of the Deaf, 1997) attaches some importance to the development of speech, but it is not expected that speech will be the primary means of communication or that verbal language will be the deaf child's first language: the development of both speech and sign language is allowed but with speech secondary to the development of sign language.

It must be asked, however, whether, with the bilingual approach, it is possible for a very deaf child to acquire speech when so much emphasis is given to sign language input. Oralists argue that, if speech is to develop, it is imperative that deaf children are given the maximum opportunity to learn to listen. If deaf children are offered a significant input of sign language in the early years, this 'easier' communication option will almost certainly be selected: their attention to the world of sound will be undermined. Since sign language is the child's 'choice', it could be argued that sign language is the child's natural language. However, those advocating an auditory-oral approach would say that it is the more 'difficult' option, of learning to listen in order to speak, that will, in the long run, offer the deaf child the greater social and educational opportunity.

Furthermore, it could be argued that, if speech is the primary goal, bilingualism for deaf individuals is still an achievable goal. It is possible to conceive of sequential bilingual development in which spoken language and sign language are the two target languages but in which the development of spoken language comes first. The auditory-oral route to bilingualism would be to develop oral communication and spoken language as a first language during childhood. The deaf child then learns sign as a second language as an older child or young person.

Many orally educated deaf adults have chosen to learn sign language and now communicate primarily through sign (Winston, 1990). It seems to be the case that some Deaf individuals, currently prominent in the Deaf community, had little or no input of sign as young children. This suggests that acquiring sign language at a later stage is a genuine communication option but not one that is acceptable within a bilingual approach.

Defining the mother tongue – whose decision?

The Deaf Community believes that sign language *is* the first language of the deaf child, and most statements made about bilingual education emphasize the importance of the role of Deaf adults in the education of deaf children (British Deaf Association, 1996; Pickersgill, 1997). Given that a hearing parent or educator cannot *really* know what it is like to be deaf, it would be difficult to argue a case against the involvement of Deaf or deaf people in the education of deaf children.

However, whether or not the Deaf Community has the right to take ownership of the decision of the deaf child's first language can be challenged. It is *not* the case that all deaf individuals choose to identify primarily, or even at all, with the cultural and social world of the Deaf (Lynas, 1994; Gregory et al., 1995). Some deaf children learn to communicate through the language of their hearing families, neighbours and schoolmates because they are encouraged to use their hearing and to talk. Yet deaf children, especially those with the greater hearing losses, who have sign language as a first language selected for them may not have the opportunity to learn to talk and socialize easily with hearing people; they may not have much choice as adults except to have a social identity as a Deaf person. A serious problem with the bilingual position thus relates to the right of some adults who are Deaf to make fateful decisions on behalf of all deaf children about their first language and primary means of communication.

Conclusion

What seems to emerge from an exploration of communication options for the deaf is a situation of uncertainty and moral dilemmas. The auditory-oral approach, although more successful in giving oral language to deaf children than in years gone by, still does not guarantee fluent spoken communication for all profoundly deaf children, nor does it offer, for some, easy communication in many situations where speech is used. However, the approach does offer speech and the ability to communicate with the rest of society, and that might be seen to be important. TC, at least as widely practised, has made little contribution to the overall raising of academic and linguistic standards of deaf children but may have a role to play in facilitating communication in some contexts and in developing communication at some stages. The bilingual option has the advantage, in theory, of offering deaf children an 'easy to acquire' language – sign language – and communication, and through signing literacy, but we do not know whether the 'in theory' goals of bilingualism are achievable for the majority of deaf children. The bilingual option has the disadvantage that speech is not a primary goal.

LEA Services in the UK are increasingly offering more than just one communication approach (Eatough, 1995), but it is not the case that all three approaches are available in each LEA area. It is therefore important that parents are on their guard against being persuaded to select an option simply to fit in with what happens to be provided within the LEA. Parents need to be aware that what is 'standard practice' in one LEA, or district within an LEA, may be unobtainable in another area. For example, in many LEAs, an auditory-oral education for profoundly deaf children is not available because *all* profoundly deaf children are believed to need sign support or sign language. In some LEAs, sign language options are not available in the local area, although they may be available 'out of district'.

It is equally important that parents are aware that there are discrepancies between the communication 'options' offered and the *quality* of that provision. That communication options are 'available' does not mean that the different approaches are being delivered effectively. The bilingual option, particularly, has very difficult and demanding requirements, and it is acknowledged by some bilingualists that this approach will fail if not properly implemented or thought through (Pickersgill, 1997). That different communication options for deaf children appear to be available should not delude anyone into thinking that what is actually on offer is necessarily a faithful realization of a particular approach.

Parents who are unhappy with the advice they receive from the professionals in their local area, or the educational practices they observe, should, in my view, seek a second opinion. If parents feel that a sign approach is being 'foisted' on them, the Deaf Education through Listening and Talking Association (DELTA) or the Ewing Foundation might be approached to offer advice. If a parent believes that the auditory-oral approach offered is not suitable for their child, the National Deaf Children's Society (NDCS) can offer a range of alternative advice.

Decisions on the selection of communication approach are determined as much by the ideas of adults as by intrinsic, unalterable features of the child. It would be so much easier if it were otherwise, if the approach selected could be dictated simply by the 'needs' of the child. The most important factor, in my view, is which of the alternative options available to the young child will be least constraining and will leave most options open to the deaf child on becoming an adult. It is this consideration which should be uppermost in the minds of those making the choice on behalf of the deaf infant.

References

Ackerman J, Sutherland H, Young A (1997) A practice report: bilingual/bicultural workshops for hearing families. Journal of the British Association of Teachers of the Deaf 21(3): 58–61.

Ahlgren I (1994) Sign language as the first language. In Ahlgren I, Hyltenstam K (Eds) Bilingualism in Deaf Education: Proceedings of the International Conference on Bilingualism in Deaf Education, Stockholm, Sweden. International Studies on Sign Language and Communication of the Deaf, Vol. 27. Hamburg: Signum Press.

Ainscow M (1995) Education for all: making it happen. Support for Learning 10(4): 147–55.

Axelsson M (1994) Second language acquisition. In Ahlgren I, Hyltenstam K (Eds) Bilingualism in Deaf Education: Proceedings of the International Conference on Bilingualism in Deaf Education, Stockholm, Sweden. International Studies on Sign Language and Communication of the Deaf, Vol. 27. Hamburg: Signum Press.

Baker C (1978) How does 'sim-com' fit into a bilingual approach to education? In Caccamise F, Hicks D (eds) American Sign Language in a Bilingual Context: Proceedings of the Second National Symposium on Sign Language Research and Teaching. Silver Spring, MD: National Association of the Deaf.

Baker C (1997) Deaf children: educating for bilingualism. Journal of the British Association of Teachers of the Deaf 21(3): 3–9.

Bamford J, McSporran E (1993) Early detection and diagnosis of hearing impairment: a United Kingdom perspective. Volta Review 95(5): 19–31.

Bamford J, Saunders E (1991) Hearing Impairment, Auditory Perception and Language Disability, 2nd Edn. London: Whurr.

Bergman B, Wallin L (1994) Swedish sign language and society. In Erting CJ, Johnson RC, Smith DL, Snyder BD (Eds) The Deaf Way: Perspectives from the International Conference on Deaf Culture. Washington, DC: Gallaudet University Press.

Bishop D, Mogford K (1993) Language Development in Exceptional Circumstances. Hove: Lawrence Erlbaum.

Bornstein H, Saulnier K (1981) Signed English: a brief follow-up to the first evaluation. American Annals of the Deaf 126: 69–72.

Bornstein H, Saulnier K, Hamilton L (1980) Signed English: a first evaluation. American Annals of the Deaf 125: 467–81.

Bouvet D (1990) The Path to Language: Bilingual Education for Deaf Children. Clevedon: Multilingual Matters.

Briggs L (1991) A polytechnic with a difference. In Taylor G, Bishop J (Eds) Being Deaf: The Experience of Deafness. London: Open University.

British Association of Teachers of the Deaf (1997) Journal of the British Association of Teachers of the Deaf 21(3). Volume dedicated to bilingualism in deaf education.

British Deaf Association (1996) The Right To Be Equal. British Deaf Association Education Policy Statement. London: BDA.

Clark M (1989) Language through Living for Hearing-impaired Children. London: Hodder & Stoughton.

Conrad R (1979) The Deaf Schoolchild. London: Harper & Row.

Cummins J, Swain M (1986) Bilingualism in Education: Aspects of Theory, Research and Practice. London: Longman.

Deaf Education through Listening and Talking (1997) The Right To Hear and Be Heard. Education Policy Document. Haverhill: DELTA.

Denton D (1976) The Philosophy of Total Communication. Supplement to British Deaf News, August 1976. Carlisle: BDA.

Eatough M (1995) BATOD Survey 1994; England. Journal of the British Association of

Teachers of the Deaf 19(5): 142–60.

Gallaway C, Woll B (1994) Interaction and childhood deafness. In Gallaway C, Richards B (Eds) Input and Interaction in Language Acquisition. Cambridge: Cambridge University Press.

Gee J, Goodhart W (1988) American sign language and the human biological capacity for language. In Strong M (Ed.) Language Learning and Deafness. Cambridge: Cambridge University Press.

Geers A, Moog J (1989) Factors predictive of the development of literacy in profoundly hearing-impaired adolescents. Volta Review 91(2): 69–86.

Geers A, Moog J, Schick B (1984) Acquisition of spoken and signed English by profoundly deaf children. Journal of Speech and Hearing Disorders 49: 378–88.

Gregory S, Mogford K, Bishop J (1979) Mother's speech to young hearing-impaired children. Journal of the British Association of Teachers of the Deaf 3: 42–5.

Gregory S, Bishop J, Sheldon L (1995) Deaf Young People and their Families. Cambridge: Cambridge University Press.

Hansen B (1990) Trends in the Progress Towards Bilingual Education for Deaf Children in Denmark. Copenhagen: Centre of Total Communication.

Harris M, Clibbens J, Chasin J, Tibbitts R (1989) The social context of early sign language development. First Language 9: 81–97.

Harrison D (1993) Promoting the educational and personal development of deaf children in an integrated setting. Journal of the British Association of Teachers of the Deaf 17(2): 29–35.

Harrison D, Simpson P, Stuart A (1991) The development of written language in a population of hearing-impaired children. Journal of the British Association of Teachers of the Deaf 15(3): 76–85.

Heiling K (1990) Education of the Deaf in Sweden. Occasional paper written for a Lewis and Clarke College (Portland, Oregon) world-wide survey of deaf education (working draft).

Hostler M (1987) Hearing aid policy with babies and young children. Journal of the British Association of Teachers of the Deaf 11(1): 8–14.

Huntington A, Watton F (1984) Language and interaction in the education of hearing-impaired children, Parts 1 and 2. Journal of the British Association of Teachers of the Deaf 8(4): 109–17; 8(5): 137–44.

Jansma S, Knoors H, Baker A (1997) Sign language assessment: a Dutch project. Journal of the British Association of Teachers of the Deaf 21(3): 39–46.

Johnson RE, Liddell SK, Erting CJ (1989) Unlocking the Curriculum: Principles for Achieving Access in Deaf Education. Gallaudet Research Institute Working Paper No. 89-3. Washington, DC: Gallaudet University.

Kluwin T (1981) A rationale for modifying classroom signing systems. Sign Language Studies 31: 179–97.

Knoors H (1997) Book review on 'Bilingualism in Deaf Education', edited by Inger Ahlgren and Kenneth Hylenstam. Journal of the British Association of Teachers of the Deaf 21(2): 53–4.

Krashen S (1982) Principles and Practice in Second Language Acquisition. Oxford: Pergamon Press.

Ladd P (1988) Hearing-impaired or British sign language users? Social policies and the Deaf Community. Disability, Handicap and Society 3(2): 195–9.

Lai M, Lynas W (1991) Communication mode and interaction style. Child Language Teaching and Therapy 7(3): 239–59.

Lane H, Hoffmeister R, Bahan B (1996) A Journey into the Deaf-World. San Diego, CA: Dawn Sign Press.

Lewis S (1996) The reading achievements of a group of severely and profoundly hearing-impaired school leavers educated within a natural aural approach. Journal of the British Association of Teachers of the Deaf 20(1): 1–7.

Ling D (1976) Speech and the Hearing-impaired Child. Washington, DC: AG Bell Association for the Deaf.

Luterman D (1991) When your Child Is Deaf: A Guide for Parents. Parkton, USA: York Press.

Lynas W (1986) Integrating the Handicapped into Ordinary Schools: A Study of Hearing-impaired Pupils. London: Croom Helm.

Lynas W (1994) Communication Options in the Education of Deaf Children. London: Whurr.

Mahshie S (1995) Educating Deaf Children Bilingually. Pre-College Programs. Washington, DC: Gallaudet University.

Markides A (1988) Speech intelligibility: auditory-oral approach versus total communication. Journal of the British Association of Teachers of the Deaf 12(6): 136–41.

Marmor G, Petitto L (1979) Simultaneous communication in the classroom: how well is English grammar represented? In Stokoe W (Ed.) Sign Language Studies. Silver Spring, MD: Linstock Press.

Mauk G, White K (1995) Giving children a sound beginning: the promise of universal newborn hearing screening. Volta Review 97: 5–32.

Newton L (1985) Linguistic environment of the deaf child: a focus on teachers' use of non-literal language. Journal of Speech and Hearing Research 28: 336–64.

Nolan M, Tucker I (1988) The Hearing-impaired Child and the Family, 2nd Edn. London: Souvenir Press.

Pickersgill M (1997) Towards a model of bilingual education for deaf children. Journal of the British Association of Teachers of the Deaf 21(3): 10–19.

Robinshaw H (1992) Communication and Language Development in Deaf and Hearing Infants. Unpublished PhD thesis, University of Cambridge.

Salander S, Svedenfors B (1993) Standardprov i svenska ht 92, ak 10 Ostervangsskolan [Standardized achievement test in Swedish, fall semester, 92, grade 10, Ostervang School]. Nordish Tidskrift for Douvundervishengen N1: 41–1.

Schildroth A, Hotto S (1991) Annual survey of hearing-impaired children and youth: 1989–90 school year. American Annals of the Deaf 138(1): 46–54.

Smith M (1997) Hearing aids. In McCracken W, Laoide-Kemp S (Eds) Audiology in Education. London: Whurr.

Stokoe W (1960) Sign Language Structure. Silver Spring, MD: Linstock Press.

Strong M (1995) A review of bilingual/bicultural progress for deaf children in N. America. American Annals of the Deaf 140(2): 84–94.

Tucker I, Powell C (1991) The Hearing-impaired Child and School. London: Souvenir Press.

Tymms P (1997) Attainment Study of Hearing-Impaired Children in the UK. Paper presented at the Annual Conference of Heads of Schools and Services for the Hearing Impaired, Hull, October 1997.

Volterra V, Taeschner T (1978) The acquisition and development of language by bilingual children. Journal of Child Language 5: 311–26.

Winston E (1990) English Use in the Deaf Community. Rochester, NY: International Congress of the Education of the Deaf.

Wood D, Wood H (1992) Signed English in the classroom, IV: Aspects of children's speech and sign. First Language 12: 125–45.

Wood D, Wood H, Griffiths A, Howarth I (1986) Teaching and Talking with Deaf Children. Chichester: John Wiley & Sons.

Useful addresses

British Deaf Association (BDA)
1–3 Worship Streeet
London EC2A 2AB

Deaf Education through Listening and Talking (DELTA)
PO Box 20
Haverhill
Suffolk CB9 7BD

The Ewing Foundation
40 Bernard Street
London WC1N 1LG

The National Deaf Children's Society (NDCS)
15 Dufferin Street
London EC1 8PD

The Royal National Institute for the Deaf (RNID)
19–23 Featherstone Street
London EC1Y 8SL

Chapter 6
Cochlear implants

JO EDWARDS AND ELIZABETH TYSZKIEWICZ

As a reader seeking information about cochlear implants for children, you may be the parent or relative of a child with a hearing impairment, a professional working with children who are hearing impaired or a student hoping to work in this field. You may be interested in cochlear implants in general or as an option for a particular child. Whatever your interest in the subject of cochlear implants for children, we hope that this chapter will provide answers to many of your questions.

Within the chapter, you will find information on:

- the children for whom a cochlear implant may be an option and what the expected benefits might be
- the process by which a child is referred to a cochlear implant programme
- the assessments carried out by the cochlear implant team
- cochlear implant surgery and its associated risks
- the post-implant habilitation process through which a child and family can be supported in getting the best from the cochlear implant.

The information and advice given will guide both parents and professionals through the cochlear implant process. It will also assist teachers of the deaf, speech and language therapists and other professionals in adapting their expertise to allow them to provide the best possible support for young cochlear implant users and their families.

Both authors are members of the Manchester Paediatric Cochlear Implant Team, which has been providing a service to children with profound hearing impairment and their families since 1991. We have considerable experience in providing assessment, information and training, cochlear implant fitting and maintenance, as well as post-implant habilitation and support. The Manchester team have worked with children of widely differing age, history of hearing loss and educational and cultural background.

The chapter is intended to describe a model of good practice in the field. Services for hearing impaired children, including those provided by cochlear implant programmes, vary in content and quality. We do not claim to have discovered how to deliver the perfect service for children with profound hearing impairment and their families, but we have learned a great deal from the families with whom we work about their needs and about the kind of service they expect from their cochlear implant team and local support professionals. It is essential that all those involved in the cochlear implant process, both families and professionals, are able to evaluate and question the procedures they are undergoing. We hope that the information provided here will enable them to do this with a good understanding of the relevant issues.

The term 'parent' is used throughout to refer to a child's principal caregiver. This might be a single parent, a couple or whoever is primarily responsible for that child's care and well-being. When discussing a child's 'local support team', we are referring to any teachers, speech and language therapists, doctors, audiologists, social workers and other professionals outside the cochlear implant team who have regular contact with the child. The 'cochlear implant team' are those professionals employed by the cochlear implant programme to provide assessment, information, training, equipment fitting, habilitation, maintenance and support to the child, family and local support team.

Who are the children who might be expected to benefit from a cochlear implant?

At present, the children considered most likely to benefit from cochlear implants typically fall into one of the following three groups:

- children who were born with a profound hearing loss and are currently under the age of 7 years
- children who were born hearing and have acquired a profound hearing loss through an illness or accident
- children who have had some benefit from hearing aids but whose hearing has deteriorated to a point at which powerful hearing aids are no longer helpful.

Parents can ask for a referral to an implant programme whether or not they feel that their child fits easily into one of these groups. The cochlear implant team will welcome the opportunity to assess the situation for them and give them all of the information that they need.

Cochlear implant technology continues to advance, and implant teams are increasingly experienced in working with children using cochlear implants. More and more children are now being assessed who might previously not have been expected to benefit from the device. A referral to a cochlear implant programme does not commit the family to anything, but it could be enormously valuable. The implant team are able to give clear, up-to-the-minute information about the cochlear implant and the children for whom it may be suitable. If, as yet, there is no accurate information about the child's hearing levels, the assessments carried out by the implant team can sometimes help to give a clearer picture of the child's hearing potential. The team may have new suggestions about the options available to the child and his family.

What is a cochlear implant and how does it work?

Cochlear implants first became available in the UK in the early 1980s. At that time, cochlear implants were only offered to adults; they have been available for children in the UK since 1988. The cochlear implant has frequently been portrayed in newspapers and on television as a kind of 'miracle cure' for deafness. Terms such as 'bionic ear' are used, giving the impression that a child receiving a cochlear implant will wake up following surgery with his hearing fully restored and instantly able to understand and use speech.

In the light of media mis-information like this, it is difficult to get the cochlear implant into perspective. A cochlear implant is a device that may help a child to cope with having a profound hearing loss. It is a sophisticated hearing aid, but it is, nonetheless, just a hearing aid. It will not turn a child who is profoundly deaf into a child who hears normally.

How the cochlear implant system works

In a person with normal hearing, the function of the cochlea is to receive sound, in the form of vibrations, and convert it into a signal that can be transmitted by the auditory nerve to the brain. The cochlea is a small structure, about the size of the nail on one's little finger. It is shaped like a snail's shell and filled with fluid. Along the length of the cochlea are rows of hair cells that act like tiny switches. When a sound occurs, the fluid in the cochlea vibrates, and the switches are triggered to send information along the auditory nerve to the brain.

For some people with a profound sensorineural hearing loss, the hair cells in the cochlea are so badly damaged that, no matter how large the sound vibration that reaches the cochlea, no useful signal is transmitted to the brain. Even the most powerful conventional hearing aid cannot provide enough sound information.

A cochlear implant is an electrical device that can do the work of damaged hair cells by stimulating the auditory nerve artificially. There are several companies that manufacture cochlear implants, but all the devices work in a similar way. They have two main components. One part is placed, by a surgeon, inside the child's head. The second part is worn outside the body like a hearing aid and is fitted about 1 month after the implant operation. The outside components (Figure 6.1) provide the signal and power that make the inside components work.

Sound is picked up by a microphone that is worn behind the child's ear. The sound signal travels down a cable to the speech processor, which is usually a small box worn on a belt or harness. The signal is processed, and a coded message about the sound is sent back up the cable to the transmitter coil, which is worn on the side of the head and held in place by magnets. Radio waves carry the signal through the skin to the inside part of the implant. The internal components of the device comprise the receiver-stimulator package, which is situated under the skin at the side of the child's head, and an array of stimulating electrodes on a thin wire that is fed down through the middle ear into the cochlea.

The cochlear implant is fitted to one of the child's ears, usually the one with least residual hearing. The other ear can be fitted with a hearing aid or left without any device. It is only worth using a hearing aid together with the cochlear implant if the cochlea on the non-implant side has some sensitivity to sound.

What is a cochlear implant programme?

Cochlear implant programmes in the UK are an NHS provision. Each cochlear implant programme employs a team of professionals, with

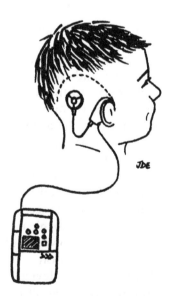

Figure 6.1 The external components of the Nucleus CI24M cochlear implant system.

a variety of skills, to provide the necessary information, assessments, equipment fitting and rehabilitation for the children and families referred to them. They occasionally differ with regard to the age of the children they will consider for assessment. Some programmes may have particular expertise in dealing with very young children or adolescents.

The parents of a child who has a hearing impairment will already be in contact with a number of health and education professionals who form their child's local support team. Referral to a cochlear implant programme almost certainly involves them with several others. Most cochlear implant teams include audiologists, teachers of the deaf and speech and language therapists. If a child goes on to have a full assessment and eventually to receive a cochlear implant, the family will also come into contact with ENT surgeons, anaesthetists, radiologists, nurses and other hospital staff. It is important that parents feel comfortable dealing with members of the team and feel free to discuss any questions or concerns throughout the cochlear implant assessment, fitting and habilitation process.

How can a referral to a cochlear implant programme be obtained, and how is it paid for?

Referrals to cochlear implant programmes are made by medical professionals, such as a family doctor, paediatrician, senior clinical medical officer or ENT consultant. Cochlear implant centres can provide information about how to obtain a referral. If there are difficulties, the child's family can of course seek a second opinion. The provision of a cochlear implant for a child is normally funded by that child's local health authority. A cochlear implant team may not be able to offer a child an appointment until they receive confirmation that this funding is available. It may be helpful for parents to contact a representative of their local health authority directly to find out what the policy is with regard to funding cochlear implants for children.

It is usually most convenient for a child to be referred to the cochlear implant programme that is closest to his home. This cuts down on the time spent travelling to and from appointments and makes it easier for members of the implant team to visit the child at school or at home, but alternative arrangements are sometimes made.

A private health insurance policy is unlikely to cover the full cost of a cochlear implant, although it may provide funding for a child to be assessed by a cochlear implant programme. If you are considering taking on the cost privately, or trying to raise money to pay for the cochlear implant, remember that the child is likely to need life-long follow-up, spares, repairs and maintenance, and may eventually become financially responsible for all of this.

What are the possible benefits and limitations of the cochlear implant?

A person who hears normally cannot listen to a cochlear implant and find out what it sounds like. However, one way of telling how much sound information the cochlear implant can provide is to look at the benefit it brings to the children who are already using the device. Amongst these children, the range of outcomes is enormous. At one extreme, there are children using cochlear implants who are able to use spoken language as a primary means of communication and to cope with a mainstream school environment with minimal support. At the other extreme, there are children who are unable to perceive or understand any sound information provided by the cochlear implant system. For most children, the outcome lies somewhere between the two.

Benefits

The cochlear implant provides access to a range of sounds. The ability to recognize and respond appropriately to environmental sounds can greatly increase a child's safety and independence. In addition, if the sound information provided by a cochlear implant is accompanied by a well-planned and delivered habilitation programme, most children can learn to understand and use some spoken language.

Factors affecting the outcome

Every child has a unique personality and an individual learning style, and this is as much the case for a child using a cochlear implant as for any other. There is no easy way to predict the amount of benefit a particular child will receive from a cochlear implant. Children differ from one another in the extent to which they are able to make use of the sound information provided by the implant system. There are numerous factors that are likely to affect the outcome for a particular child, many of which may be impossible for anyone to measure, let alone control.

Age and duration of hearing loss

Research and experience have shown that the age of a child and the duration of his hearing loss are important factors. For a child who has had little usable hearing prior to receiving his cochlear implant, the younger he is at the time when the implant is fitted, the more likely he is to make use of the device in learning to understand and produce spoken language. In children who have already had some usable hearing, consistency of hearing aid use is important. A child who has been able to make use of the auditory information provided by hearing aids will find learning with the cochlear implant easier because of his past experience of sound.

A period of normal hearing

When a child has been deafened through illness, it is important to consider proceeding with the cochlear implant as soon as possible, so that the child can attempt to 'catch up' with his auditory learning. However, recovery from all of the effects of a serious illness such as meningitis can take some time. Even if a cochlear implant is fitted quickly, it may be several months before a child is ready to begin making sense of the sound.

Listening experience

One factor that can be controlled to some extent is the kind of sound that a child experiences after the cochlear implant is fitted. Without the right listening experiences, a child finds it much more difficult to use the cochlear implant successfully. Members of the child's support team work with his family to find the best way of helping him to make the most of the cochlear implant. Besides his family, the teachers and therapists who work with the child have a vital contribution to make. Like any other child, the young cochlear implant user learns continually from the people he spends most time with, the people who take care of him from day to day.

Limitations

Using a cochlear implant should not prevent a child participating fully in a great many activities, but in choosing this device for him, we are imposing some restrictions on his life. The external equipment will probably be worn throughout his waking hours, and it is inevitable that it will sometimes be 'in the way'. Simple activities like changing his clothes, school PE lessons, hugs and cuddles may all be a little more awkward for a child who has a cochlear implant system. The cochlear implant shares many of the limitations of conventional hearing aids. The system does not perform as well in background noise as it does in quiet. A child will have difficulty hearing someone who is speaking too far from his cochlear implant microphone. He will also miss out on listening opportunities whenever his cochlear implant is not in use, i.e. in bed, in the bath or when the battery is flat or the system is broken.

The cochlear implant system can be affected or damaged by water, static electricity, magnets, a blow to the head, certain medical treatments and so on. The cochlear team can provide information about all of the limitations of the device and any precautions that need to be taken to protect it. The child comes to depend on the equipment he has been given, so that whenever any component is lost or damaged, which is bound to happen from time to time, he is likely to find life more difficult and less pleasant until his cochlear implant is functioning properly again. The cochlear implant system needs to be maintained and parts replaced throughout the child's life. Faults in the implant system are more difficult to detect and to rectify than faults in a conventional hearing aid, spares and repairs are more expensive, and, because part of the device is fitted internally, expert medical follow-up may be required from time to time.

How do the cochlear implant team decide whether or not to offer a child a cochlear implant?

The cochlear implant team need a lot of information about a child in order to decide whether the device is likely to be of benefit to him. Assessments are carried out by the team before the decision is made to offer a cochlear implant to a particular child and family. The time it takes to complete all the assessments varies.

The hearing tests

The main purpose of the hearing tests carried out by the cochlear implant team is to determine how much benefit the child is getting, or could be getting, from conventional hearing aids. The team want to know whether a cochlear implant could give him significantly more information about speech sounds than conventional hearing aids do. If appropriate, speech perception tests are also carried out. The hearing tests can take several appointments.

Speech and language assessments

There may be a formal assessment of the child's language and communication skills. Some programmes also like to see the child for a series of pre-implant habilitation sessions. This allows the team to get a clearer picture of the child's abilities and helps the child, his family and his local support team to get used to the demands of the habilitation programme.

The scan

Each child has to have a CT (computerized tomography) or an MRI (magnetic resonance imaging) scan, which is like an X-ray of his head. This allows the surgeon to look at the child's inner ear and make sure that the cochlea is properly formed and that it is possible for the electrode array to be inserted. Young children have a general anaesthetic to ensure that they lie still during the scan.

The child's history

Information about the history of the child's hearing loss and hearing aid use, his general health and development, details of his current educational programme and some understanding of his home circumstances are needed. Most of this information comes from the child's parents, but members of his local support team will also be asked to provide relevant information to the cochlear implant team.

All this information allows the implant team to work with the child's family and local support team towards the best possible outcome for that child. Choosing a cochlear implant for a child is a huge commitment, and the more honest a family can be about any difficulties they might have – with time, work, travel arrangements, expenses and so on – the easier it is to find solutions to suit their child and family. If parents are unsure why the cochlear implant team need a particular piece of information, they can ask them to explain.

Information, expectations and training

During the assessment phase, it is the responsibility of the cochlear implant team to ensure that parents have all the information that they need to decide whether to choose the cochlear implant for their child. It is essential that parents make this decision with a good understanding of the potential risks, benefits and limitations of the device. It is not always easy to maintain realistic expectations. The cochlear implant team are usually able to give parents some understanding of what the child would be likely to achieve with a cochlear implant system. It may also help parents to meet other children who are already using cochlear implants and to talk to other parents about their experiences.

Other family members, close friends, the child, his friends and members of his local support team also receive information and training from the cochlear implant team. The cochlear implant team may offer to give information seminars at the implant centre, at the child's home or at his school. They may also offer specialist training sessions to any local support professionals who work closely with the child. It is important that good communication between members of the cochlear implant team and members of the local support team is established during this period.

The decision

At the end of the assessment phase, members of the cochlear implant team discuss the results of all of the assessments, and a decision is made about whether or not it is appropriate for a cochlear implant to be offered to the child. If it is decided that the child would not receive significant benefit from using a cochlear implant, the team can offer parents advice and information about the alternatives available to their child. If a cochlear implant is offered to the child, the final decision of whether or not to proceed rests with the child's parents. If they choose to go ahead, the child will be placed on a waiting list for surgery. Providing that funding for the cochlear implant has been authorized, the child should not have to wait more than 2 or 3 months for a surgery date.

What does cochlear implant surgery involve?

The cochlear implant operation is not exceptionally complicated when carried out by an experienced ENT surgeon. Parents are usually asked to bring their child to the hospital the day before the operation and be on the ward with him for the duration of his stay. The child is visited on the ward by an anaesthetist and other hospital staff, and has some blood tests and examinations to make sure that he is well enough for the surgery to go ahead. A child with a heavy cold, a chest infection or an ear infection will almost certainly have his surgery postponed until his state of health improves. The child is not allowed any food or drink for some hours before the operation.

When it is time for the child to go to the operating theatre, his parents accompany him and stay with him until he is asleep. Once he is asleep, some hair is shaved from the side of the his head where the implant is to be fitted. The surgeon makes a cut in the skin at the side of the child's head and pulls back the skin. A shallow bed is created in the side of the child's skull in which the receiver-stimulator package is placed (Figure 6.2). The surgeon drills down through the middle ear to the cochlea. The electrode array is then fed down into the cochlea itself.

The operation normally takes between 2 and 4 hours. Parents are informed when their child is coming out of the operating theatre so that they can be there with him when he wakes up.

The child wears a large bandage around his head for a couple of days. Then, about 3 days after the bandage is removed, the stitches can be taken out. The child normally stays in the hospital for one night before the surgery and a few nights afterwards. When he returns home, he can go about his life pretty much as normal. As mentioned above, the external components of the cochlear implant system are not fitted until about 1 month after the surgery. During this time, the scar can heal, and the child's hair begins to grow back. Advice on care of the scar is given by the hospital.

Most children recover remarkably quickly from the surgery and do not seem to experience much pain, discomfort or distress. However, many parents find the sight of the bandages, scar, stitches, drips and so on quite distressing and need to be well prepared for what to expect. Surgical procedures differ slightly from programme to programme, and parents should make sure that they have details of what the surgery involves for their child from their cochlear implant team.

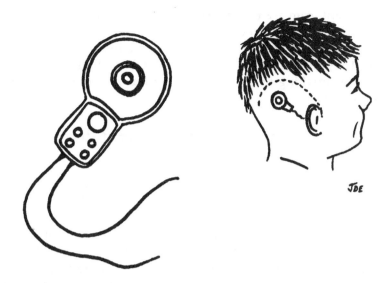

Figure 6.2 The internal components of the Nucleus CI24M cochlear implant system.

What are the risks of having cochlear implant surgery?

For most parents, the need for their child to have surgery is probably the most difficult aspect of the decision whether or not to proceed with the cochlear implant. However convinced they may become that the implant would benefit their child, the operation is always a hurdle to be surmounted. Statistically speaking, serious complications are unlikely, but statistics mean nothing if your child is the 'one in a million' whose operation goes wrong. Before the operation, hospital staff require one parent or guardian to sign a surgical consent form. Signing the consent form means that parents are accepting the risks associated with the operation and are choosing to proceed knowing that problems may arise.

Some of the risks parents should be aware of when considering cochlear implant surgery for their child relate to the general anaesthetic, the possibility of infection, device failure and facial nerve problems. It should be noted that all these are extremely unusual occurrences in UK cochlear implant surgery. Details of each risk and how likely it is can be obtained at the assessment phase from the cochlear implant team.

It is also possible (although rare) that, even with a fully functioning cochlear implant and no surgical complications, a child might be unable to perceive any sound through the device. If the child had any residual hearing prior to surgery, that hearing is likely to have been destroyed by the insertion of the electrode array into the cochlea. The child would no longer be able to receive benefit from a conventional hearing aid on that side. The other ear, however, would be unaffected.

The implant team are happy to discuss all of the risks as often and in as much detail as parents feel is necessary. If parents have specific questions about medical or surgical risks, these are best discussed with the surgeon. They should also remember to notify medical staff if they feel that there is anything in their child's medical history that might be a cause for concern.

How will we know whether the right decision has been made for the child?

Parenting involves a complex mixture of love, guilt, responsibility and worry whenever decisions have to be made on a child's behalf. There is no way of being sure that the right choice has been made for any child even in matters such as schooling, diet, discipline or medical treatment. Some of the questions that often arise for the parents of a child who may undergo cochlear implant surgery are: 'What if it's the wrong decision and makes my child ill, or unhappy, or a failure?' 'On the other hand, if I choose not to take this course, will my child feel terribly let down in later life because I deprived him of an opportunity?' Choosing to allow a child to have an operation, even though he is not ill, is enormously difficult. It is important that everyone's opinion is taken into account and that both parents agree that they want to go ahead. If at any stage a child's parents decide not to go ahead, no-one will think any the less of them for changing their minds.

Even if the decision is to go ahead with the cochlear implant, and the surgery is successful, there is always the possibility that the child will at some stage decide that he does not want to use the implant system and may question the decision that was made on his behalf. What can parents say to their child if, as a young adult, he asks why they chose to let him have a cochlear implant? There is, of course, no simple solution to these dilemmas, but we often make the following suggestions to parents on the Manchester programme:

• Take as long as you need to make the decision.
• Make sure you have collected, considered and understood every single piece of information that you need.
• Once your decision has been made, and whether or not you choose the cochlear implant, write a letter to the adult your child will become. Explain your state of mind, the information you have, why you have made your decision and how you feel towards your child. Keep it somewhere safe so that you have a record of exactly what you were thinking at that time. If, at any time in the future, your child wants to discuss the course you chose to take, you will have an honest account of it, however it turned out.

Are there arguments against the cochlear implant?

There are people, particularly those within the Deaf community, who believe that cochlear implants should not be offered to children. It is very important that those responsible for making the decision have examined all aspects of the discussion as it relates to their particular child. As well as gathering facts and information about implants and their use, parents must consider carefully the arguments presented by people and organizations who think that it is wrong for this type of intervention to be offered to children who are profoundly deaf. Information about this point of view can be obtained by talking to people at a local Deaf club, meeting representatives of organizations such as the British Deaf Association (BDA) or reading policy documents and statements from the BDA and similar national and international bodies. Information may also be available on the Internet and at the local library. Members of the local support team or the cochlear implant team can provide parents with some initial contacts.

Can the decision be delayed until the child is older?

The parents of a very young child often feel that the cochlear implant would benefit their child in the long term, but they would rather wait until he is older. Here are some of the concerns that parents may have about going ahead with the cochlear implant straight away: 'What will happen when my child's skull grows?', 'What about advances in technology?', 'Shouldn't we wait until he can decide for himself?'

For most children, whether they were born with or have acquired a profound hearing loss, the younger the child when the cochlear implant is fitted, the more beneficial the outcome is likely to be for the child's learning of spoken language. Surgeons are increasingly confident about performing cochlear implant surgery for the younger child. Children under the age of 18 months have received cochlear implants in the UK. The implanted components of the device are quite flexible and have not been found to be affected when a child's skull grows. However, it is extremely important that clear, accurate hearing test results are obtained before a child is offered a cochlear implant, and these may prove more difficult to obtain with very young children.

Cochlear implant manufacturers seem to be producing newer and better devices all the time. Parents often worry that choosing for their child to have a cochlear implant now will limit his chances of receiving a more sophisticated device in the future. The cochlear implant team offer each child the most up-to-date technology available to them at the time.

The decision cannot be delayed because, by the time superior technology becomes available, the child will have lost precious listening and learning time that can never be replaced. For the same reason, waiting until a child can decide for himself is not usually an option if he is to get maximum benefit from the device. However, if a child is already old enough to be involved in the decision, it is important for him to have his say.

Can a child who has had meningitis benefit from a cochlear implant?

Meningitis is a serious illness that can sometimes result in a profound hearing impairment. Many children who have a profound hearing loss as a result of meningitis can benefit from a cochlear implant. The implant does not restore normal hearing, but it can give the child access to sound again. A child who has had meningitis has to undergo the usual assessment procedure. However, children who have had meningitis can be regarded as 'special cases' for a number of reasons.

Ossification of the cochlea

In some cases, new bone growth can occur inside the cochleas during the weeks and months following the illness. This is known as ossification or calcification and it can make the insertion of a cochlear implant difficult or even impossible. A child who has had meningitis needs to be assessed quickly and should be referred to the cochlear implant programme as soon as a severe hearing loss is suspected. The cochlear implant team will refer him for a CT or MRI scan so that the surgeon can check for ossification.

'Fast-tracking'

If ossification of the cochlea is occurring, the child's parents may have to make a rapid decision on whether or not to proceed with the cochlear implant operation. Cochlear implant teams may have a 'fast-track' procedure for children in this situation, whereby the waiting list can be bypassed and the child offered the next available surgery date.

Having already had to live through the stress and unhappiness of seeing their child suffer a terrible illness, suddenly being thrown into this situation can be very traumatic for parents. They may have little or no knowledge or experience of hearing impairment yet are forced to try to come to terms with their child's hearing loss and comprehend the complex and difficult subject of cochlear implants. They may be asked to make a decision within the space of a few days that will affect the rest of their child's life. No-one can make this situation easier for parents, but the cochlear implant team and local support team are there to discuss with them their concerns and questions, and to help them to support their child in coming to terms with the distress and frustration of his sudden hearing loss.

How can a child be considered too old to have a cochlear implant?

A child who has had a profound hearing loss all his life will eventually be considered too old to benefit from a cochlear implant. Cochlear implant programmes differ in terms of how old they would consider 'too old' to be, but most prefer children to be under the age of 7 years when their cochlear implant is fitted. The main reason for this age limit is that research and experience suggest that a child who has not received any auditory information for 7 years or more is very unlikely to be able to learn to make much sense of the input from a cochlear implant. His brain has been busy receiving information about the world through vision, touch, taste and smell. The parts of his brain that would have been used for processing sound may have begun to process other kinds of sensory information and may no longer be available. Experience has shown that, when a child in this situation is fitted with a cochlear implant, he can find the stimulation it provides to be an uncomfortable nuisance rather than an aid to communication.

A Deaf identity

If a child is a competent sign language communicator who identifies himself very much as a Deaf person, he may feel that the cochlear implant has no place or value in his life. He may be communicating successfully with family and friends using sign language and find learning to use spoken language both difficult and unnecessary. The child may wear the implant system to please his parents and teachers but find little or no use for the information it provides.

It is still important that any child and family can get a referral for assessment by an implant team if they want one. There may be special circumstances, such as a serious visual impairment, which mean that an older child would still be considered for assessment.

Are cochlear implants an option for children with additional disabilities?

Additional disabilities do not prevent the cochlear implant being considered for a child. However, when the child's development or learning presents a complex picture, the assessment process may take a little longer. Assessments of hearing and communication may have to be modified before a clear picture of the child's situation can be established.

The outcome of the assessment phase will of course vary with the individual case. The same questions need to be answered for any child referred to the programme:

- What would the cochlear implant contribute to the child's learning?
- Will his environment give him access to meaningful auditory stimulation?
- Is the change to the child's life likely to be more beneficial than traumatic?

The cochlear implant team familiarize themselves with the child's individual circumstances throughout the assessment period. As always, it is essential that members of the child's local support team are consulted. Time must be taken to obtain a clear picture from parents and professionals about the child's personality and learning style.

Issues for assessment

It is essential for the hearing tests, and eventually for cochlear implant fitting, that a child is able to give a clear response to show that he is experiencing a stimulus. A child with learning difficulties may not yet have developed this ability and cannot be offered an implant until it has been established. A child with physical disabilities may not be able to turn towards a light or put a peg in a board in response to a stimulus. An alternative means of responding may have to be devised for the child.

Issues for management

If a child with additional disabilities receives a cochlear implant, the post-implant habilitation programme may be managed differently as there are practical issues to be considered. For example, a child who spends a lot of time seated will not be comfortable wearing the speech processor on his back. A child with a good use of one hand but a weakness on the opposite side will have the system fitted, if possible, on the side where he will be able to take it on and off himself as he grows more independent.

A child's ability to produce speech may be affected by learning difficulties or a physical disability. It is important that this issue is addressed, with help from speech and language therapists, before the cochlear implant is considered. Parents and professionals need to be clear about whether the cochlear implant is to be regarded as an aid to the child's listening and understanding or whether it is also expected to improve the child's speech production.

Realistic expectations

Parents know their own child very well and know what they are hoping for. The cochlear implant may have a valuable contribution to make to the child's situation, although the potential benefits for their child may be different from those expected for other children. With the information collected throughout the assessment period, parents should be able to form realistic expectations for their child.

When will the child begin to hear?

After cochlear implant surgery, the components of the cochlear implant that have been placed inside his head are not active. Both the power and the sound sensation will be provided by the external components of the system, which are fitted about 1 month after the surgery. A hearing aid can be worn on the side without the implant directly after surgery and, if the child gains benefit from it, together with the cochlear implant system.

The process of fitting the external components of the cochlear implant system is often referred to as 'programming', 'tuning' or 'mapping'. It is normally carried out by an audiologist on the cochlear implant team with the assistance of another team member and the child's parents. The stimulating electrodes inside the cochlea can deliver a range of sound sensations from low pitched to high pitched depending on which of the electrodes is stimulated. Programming the system involves finding the level of electrical current each electrode needs in order to provide a sound sensation to the child. The audiologist programming the device needs to know the minimum required for the child to begin to perceive a sound and the maximum that can be delivered to each electrode before the sensation becomes unpleasant. These current levels are different for every electrode of the cochlear implant system and for each individual child.

Finding out the appropriate stimulation levels for a child is like performing a hearing test. The speech processor and headset are connected to a computer that is used to play signals through the system to the electrodes inside the cochlea. The child, wearing the headset, is required to give a response whenever he perceives a sound. The kinds of response expected will depend upon his age. Very young children can learn to turn and look at a light in response to a sound. Older children may be asked to put a peg in a hole or stamp a piece of paper in response to a sound. A calm and reassuring atmosphere, the presence and closeness of parents, and amusing age-appropriate activities all contribute to the accuracy of the information obtained.

When all the channels (electrodes) have been tested and the appropriate stimulation levels have been found, information about how the implant should be stimulated is programmed into the child's speech processor. Then his cochlear implant microphone can be activated, and he can begin to hear some of the sounds around him. This may be a very disconcerting experience for a child who has had little or no access to sound prior to this moment. His reaction may be one of surprise or fear. He may be delighted with or horrified by this new experience. Whatever the child's reaction, he will rely on the adults around him, particularly his parents, to be positive and reassuring about the experience and to show him what the new sensation is for, a task that will take years of hard work and patience.

Cochlear implant programming is carried out at intervals throughout the child's life. It is normal for the levels of electrical stimulation he requires to change over time.

For the adults in the child's family and support team, what is involved before and after the surgery?

The cochlear implant team carry out a thorough evaluation of the potential benefit of a cochlear implant system for the child and inform the carers and others of how and why their decision is made. If the decision is to go ahead with a cochlear implant, a great deal will be expected of parents and, indirectly, of others in the child's life. These others include siblings, grandparents and friends, as well as, of course, members of the local support team.

There will be demands on the parents' time, with consequent effects on the time spent with the other children, partner, friends, work and leisure. There will certainly be demands on energy, and there may also be extra expenses, for example for travelling to and from the cochlear implant centre. For teachers, therapists and educational support workers, there will be modifications to the child's programme, and new training and information needs. For the adults involved, the fitting of the implant is the beginning of a long process of supporting the child in getting the best use out of it. This means a long-term commitment to keeping the implant system in good working order and to visiting the implant centre for equipment maintenance, mapping, habilitation and assessment. Most of all, the child still needs to be provided with many more opportunities to learn to communicate than are needed by a child who does not have a hearing loss.

How do the family and support team reach agreement on what decision should be made about the cochlear implant for the child?

It is important, during the assessment phase, for professionals from the local support team to discuss any issues with the child's parents, giving facts, observations and reasons in support of their comments. The child's family are likely to appreciate honesty and value the continuing support, even if doubts are sometimes expressed about the course of action they have chosen.

The cochlear implant team view the information contributed by professionals as a valuable addition to the overall picture for the child. It is important of course for local professionals to make sure that the family are aware of the content of any discussion they have with the cochlear implant team.

The decision of whether to go ahead with a cochlear implant if they are offered one reflects the family's understanding of what is best for the child. The more actively all the adults involved seek to find answers to their questions and air their views, the better informed that decision will be. The child's parents have both the right to make the decision and the responsibility for its consequences. Whatever the circumstances, the child needs consistency, positive motivation and access to education. The local support team continue to be vital contributors to his programme with or without a cochlear implant.

How can the child be prepared for the experience of having a cochlear implant?

Every member of the child's support network can become involved in the information, discussion and preparation process, including the child if he is old enough. If a child is very young and not able to partic-ipate in the kind of preparation that includes discussion, debate and questions, it is nevertheless essential to prepare him for the experi-ence of having an implant fitted, using information that is made as accessible as possible. The child is likely to feel fear and distrust if faced with the unexpected, and the information given provides both a prediction and then a record of what has happened. The ideas under-lying this careful preparation are twofold. First, the experience, although the child may not understand it, is an expected one rather than a shock. Second, as the child's understanding grows, he has a record to confirm and illustrate the possibly rather confused memories of the event.

Many different kinds of information can be used that are accessible to a child, including demonstration of the implant equipment, booklets, videos, meetings with other children, discussion and drawing with a range of different adults (grandparents, older siblings, teachers and ther-apists, as well as of course parents). Families and children also gain valu-able insights from meeting other children who use implants with their families, and talking with adult implant users.

Checking with the cochlear implant team the exact sequence of events, and obtaining any materials that they can supply, further contributes to the thoroughness of the preparation. In school or nursery, a 'hospital corner', story and picture sequences, and classroom discussion add to the picture that the child builds up of what to expect from this new event in his life. The cochlear implant team may visit his school, offer to provide resources and, if the school wishes, offer information to the child's class group.

Questions and concerns can be teased out in a variety of indirect ways, such as drawing 'before-and-after' pictures, reading stories or acting out sequences with toys. It is very important to establish what the child is expecting and also what he is afraid of. Some fears are well founded but can be dealt with quite easily ('Will it hurt?', 'Will I still be able to go swimming?'); some are equally sensible but more complex ('Will people stare at my headset?', 'Can I get rid of it if I decide I don't like it?'); and some seem absurd but are very real indeed to the child ('Will I have a wire sticking out of my head?', 'Will the doctor spill all my brains out when the operation is done?'). If a child is clearly very anxious about the idea of an implant, it is important that time is taken to get to the bottom of whatever the problem really is. A child who is not informed, and whose views are not taken seriously, may lose trust in the adults close to him if he is asked to undergo a major operation while feeling uncertain about it. He is also less likely to be an enthusiastic user of the cochlear implant system in the long term.

As a child grows older and more able to take responsibility for his equipment, he may welcome the opportunity to go back over information about how it works and is fitted, which he may have been too young to understand at the time. A photographic record in the form of an album can be a valuable resource at this stage.

From the teacher's point of view, the most vital element of the pre-implant preparation is excellent home–school communication. The teacher keeps up to date with the way in which the child's family have chosen to handle it and discusses with them the input at nursery or school. The child benefits from the reassurance of being surrounded by consistent and frequently repeated information from trusted adults.

The last aspect of preparing a child for the experience of having a cochlear implant is a word to the adults: prepare yourselves! (see the section on surgery above).

What is habilitation?

Habilitation is 'the process by which professionals support a child and family in adapting to hearing loss, getting used to a hearing device and developing the child's language and communication skills' (Manchester Paediatric Cochlear Implant Programme information booklet).

Habilitation is different from education in that adaptation to hearing loss, the good use of a hearing device and language learning (those things which make up 'habilitation') allow a child to gain *access* to education. In most areas, habilitation and education are provided by the same team of people, mostly teachers of the deaf. There may also be support from audiologists, speech and language therapists, health visitors, community paediatricians and many others. As far as the cochlear implant team are concerned, habilitation for the child involves getting the best out of the cochlear implant device and supporting its use. In order to achieve this, there needs to be co-ordination with the habilitative and educational input from the local support team.

Why is specific habilitation input needed when a child is going to use a cochlear implant?

The cochlear implant device is designed to allow users to hear sounds around them and, most importantly, the complicated and constantly varying sounds of speech. People who are new to the subject often assume that the fitting of the device automatically leads to a 'catching up' process for the child. They wonder why children who are born deaf but have implants do not begin to understand and use spoken language within weeks. It should be apparent from the information in this and other chapters in the book that the reality is far more complex where profound hearing loss is concerned.

We sometimes use the following analogy:

> As a hearing person, I cannot hear what people in Hong Kong are saying. If somebody connects me by phone to a person in Hong Kong chatting in Cantonese, the answer to the question 'Can you hear it?' would be 'Yes'. However, it would take years of listening and studying and concentration and repetition before I could understand any of it.

Many children fitted with a cochlear implant system were born with a profound hearing loss. For them, the system may be the first ever 'phone line' to speech. For children who have had some benefit from hearing aids, it may be an improved, but disconcertingly different, phone line. For children who have lost their hearing, it can be completely different from what they remember about normal hearing and at first disappointingly difficult to understand. The purpose of the habilitation work, which starts before the surgery takes place, is always to gain maximum benefit from the new equipment and become confident, skilled and purposeful in using it.

How should expectations be modified for a child who starts using a cochlear implant system?

The habilitation programme is not an 'add on' to the week's activities. It is a carefully planned modification of the child's environment, which has

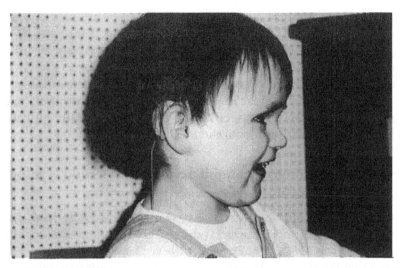

Figure 6.3 The speech processor is worn on a soft harness under the child's clothes.

to be constantly revised to take into account changing goals and expectations. In collaboration with the cochlear implant team, the starting point for the child's auditory processing and spoken language abilities must be established.

In order to plan effectively, adults imagine themselves in the child's situation and identify the auditory language learning opportunities to which he is exposed throughout the day. Which ones can be modified to take into account the new hearing potential? What receptive and expressive language goals can be selected for a particular focus within routine activities? How can other people, such as friends, mainstream teachers, dinner supervisors and nursery nurses, be made aware of the need for maximizing auditory learning? The child needs to be supported but also stimulated and 'stretched' in the use of the new device in order to benefit from its full potential.

For example, when a child can identify and respond appropriately to his name in a quiet environment when he is expecting to be called, there are other stages to move on to. Can he then tell his name from those of other children? Pick out his name against background noise? Respond when visually distracted or absorbed in a task? Respond at a distance? Locate the person calling him? Every part of the habilitation programme must be on a developmental continuum and be relevant to the learning environment and to effective communication. No 'listening' goal can stand alone as an achievement because the relevant question is not 'Is he listening?' but 'What is he learning by listening?'

Really purposeful pre- and post-implant habilitation is a process of integrating the new device into the child's life and learning. The implant's performance as a hearing device, and the child's performance at 'listening', are never the ultimate aim. The aim is to use the implant to build reliable bridges between the child and the experiences that will make his childhood as rich and exciting as he deserves. The medium for this learning is language, and the choice of an implant implies that *spoken* language is going to play a major part.

Any scheme that views '(re)habilitation' as a separate and definable activity should be viewed with caution. There is sometimes the suggestion that a child should 'do listening' for half an hour per day, a bit like a dose of medicine taken regularly to make sure that the cochlear implant will 'work'.

Contact arrangements

In addition to his home and school programme, the child may be asked to attend the cochlear implant centre at more or less frequent intervals, a cochlear implant team member may visit at home or school, or there may be a combination of these arrangements.

The professionals from the cochlear implant team are likely to include audiologists (for programming and maintenance of the cochlear implant system), teachers of hearing impaired children and speech and language therapists (for habilitative support, monitoring of progress and the essential liaison with the local support team). If the local support professionals have not previously encountered a child with a similar history and situation, the cochlear implant team offer information and training at the early stages, as well as maintaining links throughout the process of implant fitting and use.

The level of contact that the child, family and local support team have with the cochlear implant centre decreases as the child becomes a more experienced user of the system. Technical support and maintenance will always be required, however, and the implant centre should be prompt and responsive to any query about the cochlear implant system and its functioning.

What are the things to look for when setting up or evaluating habilitative support for the child who uses a cochlear implant?

Carer and child are central participants

As the child's main carers, his family are highly involved in the habilitation programme. This can be achieved in a variety of ways, for instance sessions at home, in school or at the clinic, which involve family members and the child in partnership with the therapist or teacher; carers practise skills and gain ideas for activities, follow-up and future goals; activities are designed which give a clear picture of where the child is up to and which point to where he needs to progress next; carers are supported in observing signs of progress and setting their own goals.

An outline of the habilitation programme, information about the theory underlying it and suggestions of books to read can be provided to carers and other adults supporting the child in order to allow them to be fully informed participants. Some cochlear implant programmes and/or local support teams may run parents' information meetings or training courses to enable parents to become confident and skilled in supporting their child's learning.

Short-term and long-term goals are clearly stated and understood

Short-term and long-term goals are made clear to the family members who are the child's principal carers, and they should be able to understand the link between them if the therapist explains it. Effective habilitation programmes are based on the principle that speech in real situations is the cornerstone of a child's learning with the implant system. The ultimate aim of the habilitation programme is to allow the child to work towards being able to communicate in a hearing world in the way that best suits him and his family.

It is vital that opportunities are made for discussion, collaborative goal-setting and revision. Agreed aims and regular revision of the child's individual programme should ensure that short-term and long-term goals are agreed and kept in sight by all the participants. For children of school age, incorporating these goals into the child's individual education programme is to be recommended.

Goals are closely related to everyday communication and to normal language development

Communication is a complex process, involving understanding and using language, social knowledge and speech. For a child with profound hearing impairment, it may also involve using the additional system of sign language.

If they are to be purposeful, all of the habilitation activities the child is asked to undertake should have a reasonably clear relationship to the eventual learning of communication with others. If there are doubts about the value of an activity, the adults involved can try asking themselves, 'How is this moving him closer to being able to order his own fish and chips?' If the relationship is not obvious, carers and educators ask for it to be clarified. The child has the implant as an aid to communication, and the activities undertaken are working towards that goal.

The content of the individual sessions should be highly relevant to everyday living. It should be possible to extend goals and activities to every part of the child's life: day-to-day routines at home, school life, looking at books, joining in and helping with household tasks. There needs to be close co-operation between all the people in the child's circle of family, friends and professionals to make this happen, everyone having the same high but realistic expectations at each stage. For example, if a child is going to learn to recognize and respond to his name, it is a shame for school friends or grandparents to continue tapping his arm, thereby depriving him of an opportunity to learn to use his implant. These differing expectations can be avoided through good communication between the people in the child's support network, and a good habilitation programme will put this in place. When the habilitation programme is being set up, it is helpful to establish how this is going to be achieved.

Motivation is sustained by experiencing successful communication rather than an artificial reward or extravagant praise

The habilitation programme aims to be enjoyable and meaningful to family and child, and to move them closer to the goals they have agreed with the local and implant programme habilitation teams.

The acquisition of spoken communication is a developmental process, which needs to be rewarded by success rather than excessive praise and artificial rewards. After all, if you ask for cod and chips, do you want a gold star and a round of applause, or would you rather get your supper? Communication success is a very powerful motivator and the only important one for the child's use of the cochlear implant system. For a very young child, the discovery that if you attempt to say 'more', you will receive more of what you want, is the best reward of all.

The programme is flexible and individually tailored to the child's needs

The experience of children who have normal hearing shows that learning to communicate is a gradual process starting at birth. Adults know what to expect from little children at various stages of development and can adapt their way of interacting with them without having to give it much thought. With a young cochlear implant user, things are a little more complicated. There is often a sizeable lag between how old the child actually is and the level of communication knowledge that he has.

Children all have different starting points, a variety of prior experience and individual learning styles, as well as being of different ages and abilities. Starting to use a cochlear implant represents a significant alteration to the child's experience of the world. The exact nature of the alteration depends on what the situation was before the implant. The same goals, with the same starting point, cannot be offered to all the children on a cochlear implant programme. A good habilitation programme is able to give very clear indications of where the child is up to and tailor the goals and tasks to this level.

The following examples serve to illustrate just some of the wide variety of habilitation requirements among children who are starting out with their new cochlear implant systems.

Sarah

Sarah is 6 years old and has been profoundly deaf from birth. She does not express herself through speech but is a confident and fluent user of sign language. She likes her new cochlear implant system but cannot yet identify any of the sounds she hears.

Sarah's 'hearing age' (the time since her implant was fitted and she experienced an auditory sensation) is only a few weeks even though her chronological age is 6. Sarah's habilitation programme takes into account her interests and ideas as a 6-year-old (expressed through sign), while offering her the auditory learning experiences of a very small baby (a tuneful voice, short and highly relevant spoken utterances, lots of repetition and long pauses). It includes some coaching in how to use the new hearing sensation in everyday life: which sounds it is OK to ignore (e.g. the washing machine starting up), which ones are sometimes important (e.g. the doorbell) and which ones always have an expected social response (e.g. someone calling 'Sarah'). Sarah will learn many of these new behaviours by observing other people demonstrating and explaining to her how *they* use *their* hearing. There is therefore a need for everyone around her to be involved and to give her as many learning opportunities as possible.

As Sarah progresses and acquires some comprehension of familiar items, trusted adults can use a 'speech, speech, then sign' routine to allow her to understand through speech without ever having to feel that she is being tested and can fail. There is a wide gap at the outset between Sarah's knowledge and communication ability in sign and in speech. She will continue to need stimulation and input at the appropriate level in both. This is a challenge that requires careful planning and regular review.

John

John is 2 years and 2 months old. He was born with a profound hearing loss and has used hearing aids since he was 11 months old. He has now switched to a cochlear implant system. John is a very noisy boy but does not use any recognizable words. John and his family are not using sign language and do not plan to. John has a new cochlear implant system and is wearing it for most of his waking hours, although he sometimes pulls the headset off and chews the microphone.

John is still very young and has not started his language learning yet because of his profound hearing loss. His carers can reasonably hope to take him, slightly late, through the process of spoken language learning using his implant. However, John requires enhanced input, and his carers need to readjust to his 'hearing age', which is even younger than his years. They also need to be vigilant about practical problems (e.g. pulling off the headset) and creative about solving them (e.g. showing John that he can pat and feel his headset and then bring his hand down to a toy being presented to him as an alternative). The activities and input need to take into account the stamina, interests, routine and attention span of a 2-year-old child.

The language selected for particular targeting is the highly relevant baby language of home and everyday life (e.g. 'All gone!', 'Poo!', 'Oh dear!' and 'Night night'). John's immediate and extended family and support team may need coaching and information on how to modify their interaction with him, after a year of expecting him to hear very little, and they may also need to discuss their expectations and support each other through the hard early months when John may be taking in a great deal but not saying very much. Careful thought needs to be given to compensating for the times when John does not have access to language, for example when he is in the bath.

Henry

Henry was born with normal hearing. He developed spoken language quickly and was speaking in sentences of five or six words when he became very ill with meningitis at the age of 2 years 6 months. When he had recovered, Henry had a profound hearing loss and difficulties with balance and motor control. Henry had very fleeting attention and had stopped speaking almost completely. He did not appear to have any understanding of speech. His cochlear implant system was fitted at the age of 3 years 1 month. Ossification in the cochlea means that Henry has seven active stimulating channels instead of the usual 20 for that particular system.

Although Henry has made a start using his cochlear implant system, and is clearly hearing sounds around him, the habilitation planning must take into account the fact that both he and his family are still in the process of recovering from a highly traumatic and damaging illness. It must also allow for the amount of energy and 'brain space' Henry is having to use to regain his motor abilities and contend with his impaired concentration. It is likely that Henry will continue to recover steadily in all areas over the next 2 or 3 years, and his language learning (or relearning) cannot move at a faster rate than his overall progress. Henry needs structure, clarity and consistent expectations to help him work towards regaining meaningful communication. His family have a clear and recent memory of him as a well child and need support, encouragement, short-term realistic goals and information that allows them to see even small indications of progress.

Henry's programme needs to be reviewed and revised at frequent intervals, in consultation with his family and with all the professionals in his support team (including physiotherapist, occupational therapist, paediatric neurologist and others).

The vocabulary and communication goals for Henry are based on things which were known and familiar before his illness, but are now modified to take into account his altered level of understanding.

Naomi

Naomi is 9 years and 8 months old. She was born with a moderate hearing loss and has used hearing aids since she was a year old. Naomi has acquired a good knowledge of spoken language and attends a mainstream primary school with support. From the age of 7, Naomi's hearing steadily deteriorated until, at 8, she had become totally deaf and dependent on lip-reading, at which she is very skilled, especially with familiar speakers. She has a new cochlear implant system, which she was very keen to have fitted because she wants to talk on the telephone as she used to do with her hearing aids when she was younger. Naomi cried a little, from shock, when she first heard the sound from her implant system, but now she is enthusiastically seeking auditory experiences such as the flushing of the toilet and the ringing of the telephone. Naomi can hold a fluent one-to-one conversation if she is able to lip-read but is very doubtful of her own ability to understand speech through audition. Like many children her age, she is convinced that every task or exercise has a 'right' answer and is nervous of failure.

Naomi's habilitation programme focuses on experiences designed to allow her to build up trust in her own ability to use the implant system in communication. As she has no problems with lip-reading, she does not need practice at it. However, if she is faced with challenging 'auditory alone' tasks, she may feel under pressure. Much of the work undertaken with Naomi consists of subtle modifications to her environment: her family may present familiar comments and instructions without first making sure that she is watching and then add information only if she is not sure. Her habilitationists and teachers can disguise a great deal of auditory stimulation within normal interaction and games. Adults model for Naomi the acceptability of asking for a repetition, or of asking for more information, if you do not get something the first time. This type of 'conversational repair' skill is built in, and promoted, in all activities, whether they are formal or informal. When Naomi attempts to use the telephone, structured training, with a high level of success, is offered by her habilitationist before she attempts independent telephone conversations. As Naomi learns to use her cochlear implant system, her progress is regularly discussed with her, and positive elements are pointed out. Naomi herself is encouraged to comment and feed back on how things are going for her.

Parents can make an enormous contribution if they are invited to collaborate in tailoring the programme specifically for their child. Their knowledge of their child's character, interests and preferences can profitably be sought by the habilitationists to help them design an individualized programme. The programme can undergo modification at any time in relation to the feedback they and their child provide.

Communication between the participants is frequent, clear and detailed

Communication can be established by a variety of means (a 'contact book', a videotape that is taken at the session and sent to home and school, telephone calls and regular reports addressed or copied to the carers), allowing all the members of the child's support network to receive information and to comment. Communication and record-keeping allow families to monitor precisely what is being attempted and achieved, and to follow through at home. Clarity and detail are important. Compare the following two versions of written information for parents after a session at nursery school:

We played in the water today, and Jenny really enjoyed it.

with

Water play, language used: pour it in, stop!, more, all wet, splash, my turn; listening/speech: listening for and responding appropriately to 'my turn', 'stop', and 'more', using these to cause others to perform an action; suggestions for follow up: use same language when making a drink together, washing up, giving the dolly a bath; listen for and expand Jenny's vocal attempts; show that you hear her by responding appropriately.

At the planning stage, those involved establish what sort of information will be recorded about the child's programme and how it will be conveyed to the family and to the other members of the child's support network. Close liaison is maintained between all the adults in the child's life to ensure that he is surrounded by a rich and coherent auditory and linguistic environment. 'Listening skills' practised in isolation have limited potential to ensure that the child achieves integration of the implant into all of his learning.

It is enjoyable, although it may be hard work

If any of the adults in the child's environment notices that he appears to be becoming stressed, or less willing to use his cochlear implant system and participate in activities, something is wrong. There can be no doubt of the hard work, commitment and thorough planning required on the part of the adults, but the child, if the habilitation programme is tailored to his needs, should get enjoyment and satisfaction from using and learning from the new auditory input. If the problem cannot be traced to equipment malfunction, it may be time to review the child's individual programme.

Other people can also find that they are not enjoying the habilitation process as much as they would like:

Parent: I feel guilty if I sit down to read the newspaper ... He gets fed up of me telling him to listen.

Teacher: I'm not sure if I'm doing the right things ... I can't fit it into the school day.

Sibling: Mum, you always do things with him, never with me ... Why's he allowed time off school and a hamburger on the way home?

If there is worry and stress such as is implied in these comments, it is usually possible to resolve it by reviewing what is being done, listening to everyone's comments, taking advice and making changes as needed. Do not suffer in silence!

What are the implications of the cochlear implant for the child's school?

The specialist teacher and speech and language therapist can, when a child is to have implant surgery, find themselves facing high expectations with what feels like very limited information. The child expects troubleshooting of the device and support for its use, just as with hearing aids; the child's family expect the teacher's professional expertise to encompass the necessary areas; the cochlear implant team expect to benefit from the teacher's essential knowledge of the child's home or school programme and from collaboration during the pre-surgery and post-surgery phases of the procedure; the school or nursery staff expect information and support to be available for them.

As important members of the child's habilitation and education support team, the teacher and speech and language therapist already have long-term aims and planned goals, and a routine for delivering the individual programme. Many components of this remain the same, but there will also be major modifications or additions relating to the use of a new sound perception device. As can be seen from the following sections, local support team members need information in a number of different areas.

How can the local support team obtain technical and practical information about the device: how it works, how to check and maintain it, and how to ensure that it is working to its potential?

Technical information is of two kinds. First, it is important to have general background information on implant systems, including updates on new products and technical developments. Possible sources for this are textbooks and professional journals (only recent publications being really useful as information in this field becomes obsolete very quickly), material published by implant manufacturers (often easily available on request), publications by professional or voluntary bodies, the Internet, brochures and other material distributed by cochlear implant centres, training courses and conferences. Some university training departments offer more in-depth study in the form of 'distance learning' modules, which sometimes include practical workshops.

Second, in order to provide effective support to the children in their care who use implant systems, teachers and speech and language therapists need day-to-day practical guidance on the care and maintenance of the device and on any issues specific to the particular child. This is available from the cochlear implant centre. Cochlear implant teams generally respond favourably to information from the local support team on what their particular training and information requirements are. The cochlear implant team will also approach the local team with the offer of information and to set up the collaboration that will be needed for the child to get the best out of the implant.

Some cochlear implant teams offer free professional training as part of the cochlear implant 'package' for the child, and this can be a good opportunity to ensure that colleagues also receive up-to-date information straight from the 'horse's mouth'. The teacher and speech and language therapist, who are the principal support workers for the child, are the contacts within the local service for communication with the cochlear implant team. It is helpful to them if they have a named person within the cochlear implant team to ask for if queries arise.

Can the child continue with his previous habilitation and education arrangements in school?

There is no reason to abandon any elements of the good practice in the child's programme before his implant. However, there has been a change in his situation, and consequent action is needed to ensure that this change is beneficial in the long term.

In order to integrate the cochlear implant into the child's language and education support programme, it must be viewed as a new tool to give access to sound, which requires awareness of the following principles.

The child is dependent on adults for his first auditory learning experiences

Brand new listeners do not expect a strange new signal to be meaningful and will not give much overt evidence that they hear and understand until they have been given opportunities for developing these abilities. Unless there are clear habilitation goals and explicitly changed expectations in school as well as at home, it is easy to get into this cycle of discouragement:

> *'I called him, and he didn't turn round'* ...
> therefore ...
> *'the device can't be working'* ...
> therefore ...
> *'there's no point in calling him, so I won't.'*

This then becomes a self-fulfilling prophecy because the child, having no learning opportunities, does not develop the ability to respond to his name.

The child is dependent on his equipment, and on adults to ensure that it is giving him optimal benefit at all times

It is vital to establish, and use, a quick, efficient and reliable way of ensuring that the child is perceiving the sounds that he needs to learn to make sense of. In the case of a beginning cochlear implant user, this will be a simple speech sound detection task, but as soon as possible, the child needs to give more precise feedback by identifying or imitating the sounds. Teachers and therapists must have a clearly established 'baseline' for the child's ability to do this task so that any variation will alert them to a possible problem with the cochlear implant system. The child cannot benefit from even first-class auditory input unless he is able to perceive it clearly. Any technical problems must be solved immediately, just as with other sound perception devices such as hearing aids, before proceeding with the lesson or activity.

How are liaison, support and collaboration to be organized between home, the education service and the cochlear implant centre? Whom should I contact with queries?

The assessment, fitting and habilitation protocol followed by the cochlear implant centre involves contact with the members of the local support team. The teacher and speech and language therapist may be asked for a range of information, may be invited by the child's parents to accompany them to the implant centre and will certainly have contact with habilitationists from the team once the child begins to use the implant. If a working relationship is established in the pre-implant phase, this contributes to the smooth and well co-ordinated delivery of support for the child.

Asking questions, offering information and sharing observations, records and assessment results are all much appreciated by the cochlear implant team as they put together an implant fitting and support package for the child.

There is no standard way of delivering post-implant habilitation, but it may be useful to refer to certain types of document for information about what to expect; these include quality standard documents from cochlear implant centres and related organizations, recommended practice guidelines from professional bodies and information documents from cochlear implant teams. The key to effective follow-up is, as always, good communication. This needs to be maintained in both directions, the child's family, of course, being kept in the picture at all times.

Does the fitting of a cochlear implant system mean that a child has to stop using sign language?

The cochlear implant can be viewed as an improved hearing aid for a child who has extremely limited access to sound. It should, if all goes well, add to and enrich the child's educational programme and life experience. It should certainly not be a reason to take anything away. If a child is already communicating through sign, the addition of auditory information and spoken communication offers him a choice for the future. For families who are very keen to offer their child spoken language as his primary mode of communication, the cochlear implant may give this course of action an enhanced chance of success.

It is important to reiterate, however, that, regardless of whether the child is using sign language at the time of the implant, the home and educational situation should be considered in the light of the potential auditory experiences on offer. The successful use of an implant presupposes that the user wants to listen and has the opportunity to learn to do so. If a choice has been made for the child to live and be educated in a largely silent environment, the implant will genuinely not be a useful addition and may be an intrusive nuisance. In this case, deciding *against* the implant can be a positive choice for the child.

Conclusion

A cochlear implant is a sophisticated hearing device, now available throughout the UK, which has both benefits and limitations. Establishing whether it is likely to be of benefit to a child is a complex process that must be carried out with thoroughness and extensive consultation. Informed decision-making is a high priority for the child and for all those concerned with his welfare. The authors hope that the information covered in this chapter will contribute to the fact-finding and reflection of both families and professionals faced with this still relatively new technology.

Further reading

Cole E (1992) Listening and Talking, a Guide to Promoting Spoken Language in Young Hearing Impaired Children. Washington, DC: AG Bell Association for the Deaf.

Estabrooks W (Ed.) (1994) Auditory Verbal Therapy for Parents and Professionals. Washington, DC: AG Bell Association for the Deaf.

Flexer C (1994) Facilitating Hearing and Listening in Young Children. London: Singular Publishing.

McCormick B, Archbold S, Sheppard S (1994) Cochlear Implants for Young Children. London: Whurr.

Manolson A (1992) It Takes Two to Talk, a Parent's Guide to Helping Children Communicate. A Hanen Centre publication. Bicester: Winslow Press.

Nevins M, Chute P (1996) Children with Cochlear Implants in Educational Settings. London: Singular Publishing.

Tye-Murray N (1994) Let's Converse: A 'How to' Guide to Develop and Expand Conversational Skills of Children and Teenagers Who Are Hearing Impaired. Washington, DC: AG Bell Association for the Deaf.

Chapter 7
Educational routes – ways and means

SUE LEWIS

> It was that same night that it occurred to me – Jamie would have to go to a different school to Susie. There was so much that would be denied him. How could he possibly manage? Where *would* he go to school? I'd never met a child who wore hearing aids before, not at any of the children's schools, so I knew they didn't go to ordinary schools. All I could see in my mind's eye was that film with Jack Hawkins in and the little girl Mandy and how they had wanted her to go away to school when she was still such a baby. Were schools for the deaf still like that? What went on in them? And then what would Jamie do after school? Where would he go, what would he do? What sort of jobs did deaf people have? – and there I was in the middle of the night with all these questions and no one to answer them.

Those of you who are parents may well empathize with the concerns, confusions and questions that Jamie's father felt so soon after diagnosis. Many professionals express surprise that the parents of deaf babies are so quick to voice their anxieties over their child's schooling and job prospects. Since most deaf children are diagnosed within the first or second year of life, the main thrust of support offered to families and children will be concerned with maximizing the preschool years rather than anticipating the school years. The teachers of the deaf and the audiological and medical personnel will seek to clarify the child's hearing status further, to establish hearing aids and to capitalize on the family's and the preschool child's natural listening and learning instincts in the home. They know, with their experience of dealing with many deaf children, that there is no such thing as the ideal school placement for all deaf children. Which school is right for which child is something that time rather than degree of hearing loss clarifies. The child's personality, learning style, rate of learning, social maturity and communicative and listening progress will all need to be taken into consideration, as will the strengths and weaknesses of local provision.

Jamie's parents, however, had never met a deaf child before. Jamie was now 7 months old and had just been diagnosed as having a profound sensorineural hearing loss. Until this point, they had taken for granted the ease with which he would enter and pass through the state educational system. Plans did not even have to be articulated – the assumption was that he would have a education similar to that of his sister and cousins, starting off at the local primary school, moving on to secondary school and then later, perhaps, to college or university.

The diagnosis of a hearing loss, or indeed any disability, casts doubt on such certainties as families like Jamie's struggle to realign their views of their children. Jamie's future and their ability to smooth it seem suddenly less secure. Although most parents anticipate the sleepless nights that accompany a new baby, the disruption to established routines and social lives – the nappies, the feeding dilemmas, the toddler tantrums and so on – they will not have prepared themselves for hearing aids, batteries and acoustic feedback, nor for the endless round of assessments, of clinic appointments and of visiting professionals, however personable and competent, who are suddenly intruding into their home lives. Parents who are used to being in control of their lives at home and at work suddenly feel themselves to be in dependency relationships with professionals whose expertise and help they need to understand the nature and implications of their child's hearing loss – and what the future might hold for them as a family.

Part of that future is the child's formal education, which in the UK begins during the year in which the child is 5, although most children attend playgroups or nurseries at least part time from the age of 3. This had happened for Jamie's older sister, who was now at primary school. Indeed, as soon as Jamie had been born, his parents, like many others, had put Jamie's name down on the waiting lists for the school and nursery of their choice to be 'sure of a place' at their local, highly respected state primary school. Now such actions appeared presumptive as a multitude of questions went through their heads:

> Did deaf children still go away to special schools?
> Did any deaf children go to their local schools?
> If they did, how did they manage if they couldn't hear?
> How would the other children and teachers react to Jamie?

Earlier chapters have explored many issues in relation to the nature of hearing loss, its early management and the ways in which the partnership between parents and professionals can support the deaf child's development. This chapter is particularly concerned with the special educational needs that deaf children might have once they reach nursery or school age, the provision that is made for them and the legal framework that underpins this. Although the examples provided will relate specifically to provision within the UK, the dilemmas and issues raised are universal.

This chapter will explore four main areas: the special educational needs that might arise as a result of deafness; the various forms of educational provision made for deaf children and the advantages and disadvantages of each; the rights and responsibilities that families have in relation to their child's education within the context of the law in the UK; and what parents can do if they are in dispute with the local authority over the most appropriate school for their child or the level of support and resources to be provided. The chapter does not seek to provide the definitive text on each of these areas; instead, we wish to raise some of the questions to be asked and point readers towards other reading or avenues of support should they require further help and information.

What constitutes special educational needs?

The 1993 Education Act defines a child as having special educational needs (SEN) if:

> he or she has a learning difficulty which calls for special educational provision to be made for him or her.

A child has a learning difficulty if he or she:

(a) has a significantly greater difficulty in learning than the majority of children of the same age
(b) has a disability which either prevents or hinders the child from making use of educational facilities of a kind provided for children of the same age in schools within the area of the local authority
(c) is under five and falls within the definition of (a) or (b) above or would do if special educational provision was not made for the child.

(Education Act 1993, Part III, Section 156)

In January 1997, 18% of pupils in England and Wales were identified as having special educational needs, i.e. were on schools' Registers of Special Educational Need (Schools Census, cited in DfEE, 1997). This concurs with the estimates in the Warnock report (DES, 1978), and in the 1981 and 1993 Education Acts, that up to 20% of children will have special educational needs at some point in their educational career. Currently, 3% of all school-aged children (DfEE, 1997) have special educational needs that are considered significant enough for a

Statement of Special Educational Need (SEN) to be issued. The percentage of pupils who do have such Statements (or Records of Need in Scotland) varies, however, from local authority to local authority. Published figures indicate that in some LEA areas, fewer than 2% of pupils have Statements, whereas the figure is over 4% in a number of others.

It is important to recognize that deafness itself does not constitute a special educational need. Special educational needs may arise as a result of deafness, however, and these needs must be appropriately provided for in order to enable a child to achieve his or her potential. A hearing loss of any degree is a potential hindrance or barrier to learning, but children with similar hearing losses will not necessarily have the same severity of need. Not all deaf children will have a Statement of SEN. Some deaf children will have their needs provided for very effectively without a Statement, and this is in line with recent DfEE guidance (1994, 1997)

Deafness and special educational needs

The impact of deafness on children's language and communicative development is well documented (see Chapter 5 for an exploration of this subject). Since most Western education is conducted through the spoken and written word, albeit in conjunction with practical experience, any linguistic and communicative delay will impact on deaf children's full access to the curriculum and to the everyday life experiences that their peers take for granted. The 1988 Education Act protects all children's right to a broad, balanced and relevant curriculum, including the National Curriculum in place within England, Wales and Northern Ireland. It follows that deaf children's continued progress in understanding and using language and in listening to learn must be supported and provided for throughout their educational career if their entitlement to such a curriculum is to be safeguarded.

A shared vision

A major factor in the ultimate decision of where Jamie should go to school will be the identification and agreement by parents and professionals of his needs and the ability of one placement, rather than another, to provide effectively for them. Where parents and professionals find themselves in dispute about a placement or about resources to be provided for a child, it may well be because they have different vantage points, with regard to not only the child's current needs, but also the ultimate objectives for him. Thus, for some parents, the need for their child to be maintained within the family and local community may far outweigh any other considerations. Other parents may feel strongly that their child needs to be taught alongside other deaf children by teachers who are qualified teachers of the deaf. Such prioritization of need will obviously drive their views on the best placement for their child: the local mainstream school in the first example, a specialist school for the deaf in the latter.

Teachers of the deaf, mainstream teachers and educational psychologists may well have visions different from those of parents; in particular, they will be influenced by their existing convictions on what the 'needs' of deaf children are and the objectives that should be set for them. These may or may not be appropriate for *this* deaf child in *this* family. Preschool programmes that have family-centred orientations (Winton and Bailey, 1994) acknowledge the skills of being able to share expertise and knowledge with families without imposing opinions or decisions. They recognize that, in the final analysis, parents retain the responsibility for their children and should be the decision-makers.

Establishing the needs

A detailed assessment of Jamie's strengths, weaknesses and needs will inform any placement decision that is made for him. This assessment process begins soon after diagnosis, when a range of 'baseline' measures are carried out against which his current and future progress will be measured. The importance of assessment to inform planning and educational programmes is recognized in the DfEE Code of Practice (1994). How and where such ongoing assessment of need takes place is not as critical as that it should take place. Some deaf children attend an assessment centre for a block of time to allow intensive observation of them as learners. Others are assessed at home and in more everyday contexts. A range of assessments may be carried out: language assessments, video analyses and observations; developmental checks of physical, social, emotional and play development to provide a broader picture. A number of professionals will be involved, particularly if the assessment is part of the local authority's statutory assessment of special educational need, to which the law requires a number of key personnel to contribute. Parents themselves are important contributors to the assessment process and have a central role to play in gathering and presenting information, in commenting on others' assessments and in identifying needs.

Hearing loss is significant not only because of its impact on communication with others and the child's ability to express ideas. Hearing is also an alerting sense: it lets us know when something is about to happen or is happening. We might then take a decision on whether to look or not, to be involved or not, to reflect on the experience or not. It follows, then, that deaf children may have a more limited range of experiences simply because they do not overhear or notice something happening. They do not have such ready access to the second-hand experiences of others through overhearing and overseeing other people's conversations. There may well be needs to be provided for that relate to this broader experiential deficit, a deficit that impacts on children's knowledge and understanding of the world, of social relationships and values, as well as on their linguistic level.

There is also a need to support Jamie's effective use of residual hearing in varying listening environments with appropriate and working amplification packages, including hearing and radio aids (FM systems) and headphone listening opportunities. Adequate classroom acoustics, as well as quiet listening conditions in a withdrawal room, will be necessary to support the further development of listening skills. Teaching needs will include support from qualified teachers of the deaf and from trained support assistants, as well as a teaching and learning environment that understands the deaf child's needs and is committed to meeting them within the context of the particular educational setting. Personal and social needs may include a need for social interaction with and opportunities to work alongside hearing and/or deaf children, to develop a positive self-image, to have opportunities for independence, to share in local community activities and so on. Curricular needs will include full and equal access not only to the curriculum in school, but also to the school's extracurricular experiences.

Individual children may have very specific individual needs, some of which will be influenced by decisions already made for them. An auditory-oral child, for example, will need to be educated in a sign-free environment; a child who uses British Sign Language (BSL) will need to be supported by individuals fluent within that language and will need peers and role models with whom he can communicate and converse. Some children may have very specific additional language and speech needs, and require an intensive and structured language programme. All deaf children will need to be in an environment that allows them to grow as individuals, to offer their own ideas and conclusions and to develop independent learning behaviours. Although they will need the support of their families and teachers, particularly in the early stages, for explanations and information, care must be taken that there are sufficient opportunities for deaf children to think for themselves. The aim is that they access the curriculum and speak increasingly for themselves rather than be dependent on others to do this for them.

Providing for identified special educational needs

The starting point for consideration of any placement for Jamie will be whether the LEA can provide for all of his identified needs within their mainstream provision. If his parents or the authority have any doubts about this, a unit or school for the deaf will be considered. If Jamie's parents have a strong wish for a school for the deaf or indeed for one mainstream placement, whilst the LEA favours an alternative, they must demonstrate how it will provide for all of his needs. Most authorities do have a very small number of pupils who attend schools for the deaf; *which* school and *which* child will depend on the child's identified needs and the school for the deaf best fitted to meet them.

Jamie's parents, when they visit the various school options for him, will want to know whether each can make the provision necessary to provide for his needs, i.e. support his social and emotional well-being, continued communicative progress, learning and academic attainment. They will want to discuss what they have seen and read with others – parents of older deaf children, young deaf people themselves, peripatetic teachers of the deaf, voluntary agencies. All will help to inform their views on the right initial placement for Jamie.

The notion of an 'initial' placement is an important one to bear in mind. Deaf children's needs do not remain the same throughout their educational career, nor does a school's ability to provide for those needs. Some children may need the intensive initial boost to their language base and learning attitude at the beginning of their school career that a unit placement or a school for the deaf specializes in providing. Others may not. A need to increase levels of support, including the possibility of transfer to more specialist provision, may be suggested at any point in Jamie's educational career if his progress is thought insufficient and he is in danger of underachieving. A transfer from a school for the deaf or unit to a mainstream learning environment may also be suggested. No placement should be regarded as permanent.

The current system of regular reviews for children with special educational needs should ensure that Jamie's parents know why a particular provision is being considered, what the school is aiming to achieve with their child, whether this complies with their own views and expectations ... *and* whether the placement is working.

Within the UK, the concept of special educational needs as defined in the Education Act is one which is clearly related to the provision that must be made to cater for such needs. For a child over the age of 2, this involves educational provision 'additional to or different from the educational provision generally made for children of the child's age in maintained schools in the area'. In the case of a child below the age of 2, special educational provision involves 'educational provision of any kind.' (Education Act 1993, Part III, Section 156)

Since local authority services for deaf children, and indeed their provision in mainstream schools, differ considerably, what is 'generally' provided in one area may differ from that in another. Nonetheless, there are some aspects of provision that will need to be protected for all deaf children, regardless of where they live. A need for effective amplification to support listening skills requires that the child has access to working hearing aids, appropriately set, and to adults who can help him check and maintain them through an effective checking routine. Such checks will include daily listening checks and regular electroacoustic testing with a hearing aid test box. There should be ongoing evaluation of the child's hearing levels, including testing the child with his hearing aids (or cochlear implant) in place, to ensure that the aids and the internal settings continue to be the most appropriate for the child's hearing loss and listening needs. The school and/or parents will need access to spare hearing aids and components. Large-group and small-group listening conditions may require the child to be provided with a radio or FM system (see Chapter 3) and a conference microphone; TV and computer adapters may be necessary. Some pupils will need the wide-band listening experiences and quality of sound that headphone listening via auditory trainers or group hearing aids can deliver. The provision of all such equipment will need to be backed up by staff who have had training in checking and using it. Intensive auditory training programmes may be appropriate, necessitating withdrawal to a quiet listening room. Classrooms may need acoustic treatment with carpets, curtains and other materials to help cut down on reverberation and background noise.

The support that will be provided to promote the child's continued linguistic and communicative progress should be outlined, including the approach to communication felt to be most appropriate and the arrangements (small group, individual and class teaching) that will facilitate the child's language acquisition and access to the curriculum. This may involve structured language programmes, conversational support work, support for thinking skills, story-telling programmes, a particular approach to reading and writing, detailed assessment and videotape analysis of the child's linguistic progress and so on.

Other special educational provision will detail the amount of support that the child will receive from a teacher of the deaf and any additional help that will be given by support assistants or mainstream subject teachers. Mainstream teachers and support assistants will need ongoing advice and training, and the specific arrangements made for this – who will do it and when – form part of the special educational needs provision made for a particular child. Regardless of whether a deaf child is being considered for a Statement or Record of SEN, the process of identifying need and monitoring and evaluating progress is an essential component of the preschool years. Ultimately, it will inform how Jamie's parents and teachers look at possible school placements and will help to clarify what each placement must offer and do to meet his needs.

Educational provision for deaf children in the UK

Within the UK, there is a range of placements available for deaf children, although not all are available in a given geographical area. Severely and profoundly deaf children attend specialist day and residential schools for deaf children, mainstream schools, specialist units or resource bases, or their local mainstream school. As for most groups of children with special educational needs, there has been a tendency over the past 20 years for increasing numbers of deaf children to be educated in mainstream settings and a resultant decline in the size and number of schools for the deaf. This is only partly linked to changes in educational thinking. Earlier diagnosis, the introduction of preschool and family support programmes, the growth of peripatetic and support services, technological advances in hearing aid and FM technology, more detailed understanding of the language acquisition process and how best to support it have all contributed to today's deaf children having a more effective base from which to learn in mainstream classes than in the past.

Current educational thinking, law and guidance are committed to the mainstreaming or inclusion of children with special educational needs (Education Act 1993; DfEE, 1997). The concept of 'mainstreaming' or 'inclusion' is an international concept. The Salamanca statement on special needs (UNESCO, 1994) calls upon all governments to 'adopt as a matter of law or policy the principle of inclusive education, enrolling all children in regular schools unless there are compelling reasons for doing otherwise'. Such an education is seen as the most effective means of not only combatting discriminatory attitudes, but also providing for the fullest educational progress and social integration.

In the UK, a number of government policy documents and discussion papers, including 'Excellence for All Children' (DfEE, 1997), reflect this position, i.e. that there are strong educational as well as social and moral grounds for educating children with special educational needs with their peers. Since the ultimate purpose of provision for the deaf child is that he should 'flourish in adult life' and 'be part of the broader community' (DfEE, 1997), an education within such a community would seem to be appropriate. However, not all professionals, parents and deaf people themselves believe this. Some deaf people believe fiercely that deaf children should be educated in schools for the deaf in preparation for life in the Deaf community (Fraser et al., 1996). The 'Standard Rules on the Equalisation of Opportunities for Persons with Disabilities' (United Nations, 1994), whilst reiterating the general principle of equal opportunities and rights for pupils with disabilities in integrated settings, acknowledge that there are situations in which 'special education' may be appropriate and that

'owing to the particular communication needs of deaf and deaf/blind persons, their education may be more suitably provided in schools for such persons or special classes and units in mainstream schools' (p.25).

In the UK, alongside the conviction that 'we want children with SEN to be educated in mainstream schools wherever possible' is a recognition that there will be a 'continuing need for special schools to provide ... for a very small proportion of pupils whose needs cannot be fully met within the mainstream sector' (DfEE 1997).

Under the 1993 Education Act and the Code of Practice (DfEE, 1994), LEAs have a qualified responsibility to provide for children's special educational needs within local schools unless this prejudices the education of other children within the school or the efficient use of resources, or is inappropriate for the child's needs. LEAs must also, however, provide information to parents not only about their own provision, but also about independent and non-maintained specialist schools, in this case for deaf children.

Severe and profound deafness is a low-incidence disability. Some smaller or more rural LEAs are finding it a challenge to cater within their own local provision for the identified needs of all their deaf children. Most do have provision to support the inclusion of deaf children in mainstream schools, either through peripatetic support from teachers of the deaf or attendance at a unit or resource base for deaf children. Very few authorities maintain their own school for the deaf, however. Many of the larger schools for the deaf are non-maintained schools, i.e. they are charitable foundations that work in close co-operation with LEAs but are independent of them. Given the small number of specialist schools for the deaf and their differing specialisms within the field, if a child needs to attend one, he may well have to board. Parents are sometimes able to move closer to the school so that the child can attend as a day pupil, an option not always practical or desirable from other family members' points of view.

Local mainstream placements

Children with special educational needs are now regarded as an essential part of the school community, with the same rights and entitlements as other children to the environment and support that they need for learning. School governors have certain responsibilities placed on them to overview the provision for pupils with special educational needs and to report on this to parents. All schools have policies for special educational needs and designated special needs co-ordinators. All teachers will have some children with special educational needs, including possibly a child with a Statement of SEN, in their classes and are expected to plan their lessons taking the needs of these children into account. Most will also be used to working with support services and to planning, implementing and reviewing individual education plans (IEPs) for pupils with special educational needs, although the school's experience of children with significant hearing losses may be limited. All schools will have been inspected under the Schools Inspection Act 1996, and parents should request a copy of their most recent report (their OFSTED report). This, in conjunction with visits and discussions with other parents, should give some insight into the school's commitment to its pupils with special eductional needs and the progress and attainments of such pupils.

There are obvious advantages to a mainstream placement for a child like Jamie – social, academic and linguistic. He would attend his local school, play and learn with local friends and grow up alongside them as part of the local community. Expectations of his behaviour, academic expectations, the curriculum taught and learning experiences provided would be similar to those for all children. Jamie would be surrounded by full and natural language, and experienced language users who are essential for his continued linguistic growth.

A mainstream education does not, however, remove the barriers to education associated with deafness. Many deaf children need considerable support beyond that 'normally' available in the mainstream school to ensure that they genuinely do have access to the 'strengths' of the mainstream school and do indeed thrive there.

Peripatetic or support services for the deaf have a long experience of supporting individual children in their local schools and an increasing experience of supporting severely and profoundly deaf children there. Deaf children with all degrees of hearing loss and levels of need do have their needs met very effectively in mainstream schools, but there are large variations in their attainments (Powers, 1996). Such variations have led some (Lynas et al., 1997) to propose that the support available is a critical factor in such attainment, and a number of research projects are currently exploring this. Most parents of deaf children, whilst at ease with the concept of their child attending a local school, are naturally concerned that the right amount of extra help, expertise and specialized equipment is in place to meet their child's special educational needs.

The support services and resources available to help to provide for deaf children's needs in local schools differ considerably from area to area, as does the attitude to mainstreaming, particularly for those deaf children like Jamie who have profound hearing losses. In some LEAs, deaf children who need extensive support from teachers of the deaf and/or other trained personnel have been traditionally placed in a specialist unit or school for the deaf rather than being maintained locally in their mainstream school.

If Jamie were to attend his local school, he might need multiple weekly visits from a qualified and experienced teacher of the deaf to his school, not simply for direct teaching, but also to plan with and train staff, to monitor learning experiences, to assess Jamie's progress, to check his amplification and so on. When deaf children are placed in their local school, the mainstream class teacher delivers the vast bulk of curriculum, but a major part of the teacher of the deaf's role will be to ensure that the educational environment in the classroom is supportive to language development and allows the deaf child access to the curriculum. The teacher of the deaf will also teach Jamie individually to move his personal, learning, linguistic and literacy skills forward. Trained nursery nurse or support assistant time may be allocated to facilitate specific aspects of Jamie's needs being met – in small-group or individual learning experiences or in the class itself. Where children use a sign support system or a sign language, a communicator or interpreter may be provided. The responsibility for the deaf child's education rests with the mainstream school and teachers, unlike in the specialist school or in some units, where the teacher of the deaf may play a major role in delivering the curriculum.

The theoretical advantages of a mainstream place, or indeed any of the placement options concerned, should not blind us to the fact that there is no such thing as the ideal placement for all deaf children. The key question concerns not whether Jamie will be able to 'manage' or 'cope' in the mainstream school but whether the conditions and resources exist in that school to support his learning and attainment. If they do not, will any additional resources provided be sufficient to do so?

Specialist units or resource bases

Most LEAs do make some provision for the needs of deaf children within mainstream schools that have units or specialist resource bases, an arrangement whereby extra resources, training and equipment, including the services of one or more teachers of the deaf and other trained personnel, are based at a mainstream school. The size and organization of such provision varies considerably, however, as indeed does the 'title' of the provision.

Powers (1990) identified 26 variations in the official titles of such specialist provision within ordinary schools. Most had the word 'unit' or 'resource' in their title but differed in whether they were a 'centre' or a 'base' and whether they catered for 'hearing impaired', 'deaf' or 'partially hearing' children. It cannot be assumed that a similar title represents any similarity in organization, philosophy or size.

The range of resources, numbers of teachers of the deaf and trained support personnel that are located on unit or resource bases vary considerably, but there will usually be at least one qualified teacher of the deaf. Additional facilities should include a quiet withdrawal base and some attention to the acoustic conditions in mainstream classes. The audiological resources, support and expert knowledge available should be greater than that available to the child in the local neighbourhood school, and, although the bulk of the child's learning will usually still take place in mainstream classrooms, some aspects of the curriculum may well be delivered by the teacher of the deaf. The teacher of the deaf will still have a major advisory and training role with mainstream teachers, but mainstream teachers and children will be very used to deaf children being part of their classes. Close co-operation between unit and mainstream staff in planning and evaluation will be necessary to ensure that there is continuity in curriculum areas, expectations and standards as well as support for the child's specific listening, learning and language needs in both mainstream and unit lessons, as the child moves between both. Deaf children think of themselves as being part of Class X rather than as a 'unit' child. They will also have two peer groups – the one hearing, the other a much smaller group of hearing aid wearers who also attend the school.

Many mainstream staff in such schools have very effective teaching skills that actively support the inclusion of deaf children in their classes. They also develop keen understandings of the specific learning needs of deaf children, use audiological equipment with confidence and draw well on the expertise of their specialist colleagues. Not all units, however, operate on an inclusive model. Some deaf children do spend the vast majority of their day in the unit classroom. In such provision, real opportunities for both academic and social integration may be very limited and often highly contrived, even if the level of specialist teaching and support available in the resource base is high. Where the children do integrate, some mainstream class teachers have been known to refuse to have a deaf child in their class if there is no in-class support available; others may not plan any support materials and activities for the child, seeing that as the unit's responsibility.

There may, of course, be very valid reasons why some individual children should spend the majority of their day within the unit context. Most children's withdrawal and inclusion timetables are indeed individual to them. It is important, however, that they are determined by 'need' and not, as in some instances, by the availability of staff, by traditional working practices or because of an attitude that sees provision for deaf children as an extra responsibility for the school rather than an integral part of it.

Deaf children cannot be said to be succeeding in mainstream education if they are socially isolated and lack confidence, however well they are doing academically.

Jamie's parents will want to investigate the way in which the units in their LEA are organized, the levels of support that will be provided and the ways in which children's inclusion in the school is ensured. A school's last OFSTED report and the school, unit or support services' prospectus will give some indications of the levels of support provided, of how the school and unit staff work together and of the attainment and progress of the deaf children based there. They will also want to know about the levels of attainment and progress of children who have gone through the unit system and what they achieve by school-leaving age.

Specialist schools for the deaf

Deaf children attend specialist schools in the UK for a range of reasons and not simply because it is their parents' wish. Although the right of parents to 'choose' which school their child should attend is protected in law, the rights of parents whose children have Statements of SEN are not so defined. Deaf children who are being considered for a specialist school placement will undoubtedly have such a Statement or will be being assessed for one. Their parents may express a *preference* for a school for the deaf, but this does not mean that the LEA will comply with this preference, although it must take it into account.

There are currently approximately 40 specialist schools for the deaf in the UK, many of which specialize in supporting deaf children with particular learning needs who need a particular approach to language acquisition and communication, and who are of a particular age or ability range. Most of these schools are small – with fewer than 60 pupils on their roll – although the largest, including a specialist grammar school for deaf children, may have rolls of over 100.

Local authority and non-maintained schools for the deaf, like other schools, are subject to inspection under the Education Act 1997 and the School Inspection Act 1996. They will have a recent inspection report identifying the strengths and weaknesses of the school and the qualifications and National Curriculum levels that their pupils have achieved. Copies of these reports and schools' prospectuses will provide an initial starting point for exploring standards and emphases. All will have a declared communication and language acquisition support policy. All should offer a range of support and provision over and above that which would be available in a local school or resource base. This should include smaller classes, a better acoustic environment, a range of audiological equipment and services, and the amount of individual and small-group teaching time available from a qualified teacher of the deaf. All staff, including clerical, care and support staff, should have had training in deaf awareness and the language and communication approach used in the school. A deaf peer group and role models should be available to support the child's broader social needs, self-image and identity.

Issues to consider and questions to ask

If the expectation is that most deaf children will attend their local school or one with a specialist resource base, when should a specialist school placement be considered for a deaf child? What are the advantages and disadvantages of the varying forms of provision made? What follows below is a brief exploration of the issues to be considered and key questions to be asked in relation to a specialist school, resource base or mainstream placement if parents and professionals are to be satisfied that it will effectively provide for a specific child's needs. These topics fall into four main areas: communication issues; teaching, learning and curricular issues; personal and social issues; and 'partnership with parents' issues. In addition, for the specialist school, there will be residential issues for those parents whose children have no option but to board.

Communication issues

This is not the time to revisit the arguments for or against the different approaches used to support deaf children's language acquisition and communication (see Chapter 5). Parents will already be using a particular approach to language acquisition with their children and will wish to have a school placement that continues to extend their child's linguistic skills within this approach. However, this may not be available for them locally at all phases of their child's education or with sufficient levels of support. All children need to be surrounded by full and fluent language in order that their own language skills and understanding move on. Some smaller authorities may be unable to provide the inputs, peer groups and role models that facilitate this within all approaches to communication and all possible placement options. They may have very effective provision, for example, for pupils who require sign support but no specialist facilities for auditory-oral or bilingual pupils. Other authorities may have strong auditory-oral provision but only limited support for the small number of pupils who require, or whose parents have opted for, bilingual or sign support provision. Parents and the LEA may then have to consider a specialist unit in a neighbouring authority or a school for the deaf that specializes in educating deaf children using the particular communication and language support approach concerned.

A number of specialist units and a smaller number of schools for the deaf aim to offer support for both auditory-oral children and those who use sign support and/or bilingual approaches. There is some debate over the appropriateness of providing for children with very different communication needs within the same educational environment. Such 'mixed' provision is increasingly part of local authority provision and certainly enables some LEA resources to be more efficiently used. Whether it is the most effective way of meeting deaf children's needs is another issue. Some parents and professionals feel very strongly that this is not what they wish for their children. They point to the rights of all children to have conditions for learning that are optimal for them (DELTA, 1998). This would include an environment committed to the language acquisition approach that they are using. For auditory-oral children, this means a sign-free environment; for those whose parents have opted for sign support or bilingual approaches, this means an environment which gives clear messages as to relative value and emphases placed on sign and spoken language. Parents who have opted for an auditory-oral approach are often particularly unhappy with such arrangements, which they feel effectively limit the local options now available to them if their child's future listening and linguistic progress is not to be compromised (DELTA, 1998).

Thus important questions for Jamie's family to ask of all types of provision they visit will be:

- What is the approach to language acquisition used?
- How will language acquisition be supported?
- Is it the same approach that we wish to be used with Jamie?

A central feature of Jamie's provision will be the continued monitoring of his linguistic progress, including his literacy development. There should be careful analysis of the adequacy of his current level of language functioning for curriculum access and clear targets set for linguistic and literacy progress at each annual review. It is usually the teachers of the deaf who carry out the linguistic analyses and advise on appropriate targets and programmes for the child. Some deaf children need access to a speech and language therapist who understands the communication approach used with the child. Most schools for the deaf and some unit provisions will have speech therapists based at least part time at the school to work with children as appropriate. This is less common in the mainstream school, where such support, if necessary, may well have to be arranged after school. Further questions relating to this area for Jamie's family are:

- How is linguistic progress assessed?
- Will specific targets be set for Jamie in this area?
- How will progress towards these be evaluated?
- How fluent are the children's communication skills when they leave school?

The importance of high levels of literacy in today's society cannot be overestimated, despite its technological bent. Much research also demonstrates that reading standards amongst deaf people are highly variable (see Chapter 5). In the mainstream, the teachers of the deaf will have a clear role to play in advising on the approach to reading and writing that will be most suitable for children like Jamie who will bring delayed – or, in the case of a BSL child, possibly different – skills to the task. This is particularly important as the government introduces the National Literacy Strategy, a major literacy initiative for schools. In the specialist units and schools for the deaf, there should be a clear indication of how they are working within such initiatives to improve levels of literacy in their provision and the approach to literacy that they are using. Important questions here are:

- What is the approach to literacy used in the school?
- How are parents involved in this?
- How does the school measure children's reading and writing progress?
- What are the overall standards of literacy like by school-leaving age?

Teaching and curricular issues

Some deaf children have an identified need for extensive teaching and support from a qualified and experienced teacher of the deaf, experienced in delivering the National Curriculum and in promoting deaf children's broader language, listening, learning and personal and social development. Currently, all teachers working in specialist schools for the deaf and units attached to ordinary schools must have a double qualification as a teacher and as a teacher of deaf children. This requirement is under review but is as yet mandatory.

The majority of teachers working within specialist provision for deaf children and as peripatetic teachers will be qualified and experienced teachers of the deaf with extensive experience of catering for the needs of deaf children, but not all are (British Association of Teachers of the Deaf, 1995). Some will be teachers of the deaf in training, and if the deaf children they are teaching have a Statement of SEN requiring specifically that they are taught by a *qualified* teacher of the deaf, the Statement is not being met. LEAs and schools will be asked what steps they will take to address this.

Most deaf children do receive high-quality and effective teaching and support from their teachers and others, as evidenced in the judgements made about quality of teaching when OFSTED teams inspect such schools. Occasionally, however, parents report their disappointment when they realize that this has not been the case:

> I heard that Mrs S. was leaving and so I asked why – expecting to be told she had another job or was pregnant or something – then they said that she had failed her course! I hadn't the slightest idea that she wasn't qualified. The school is a long way away, and D. has to go in a taxi. Twice I had said I felt D. wasn't making progress at the moment – she seemed to be doing more of the same work but not a lot that was different. Mrs S. insisted that she was doing well – was one of the best – and D. seemed happy, so I felt reassured. Now I feel terrible. D. was in her class for 3 years, and all that time

she was being taught by someone who they decided in the end wasn't a good enough teacher of the deaf! I rushed up to the school to find out which teacher she would have next – and had her other teachers of the deaf been qualified? – and no they hadn't all been, though the others had all passed their training. I liked Mrs S., that wasn't the problem – I just feel that the school should have been more honest. I keep wondering how much time she has lost. It's really shaken our confidence in the school. I mean, she went there because she needed to be taught by teachers of the deaf – that was the whole point.

In the specialist school, Jamie's parents will want to ask:

• Will the class teacher be a qualified teacher of the deaf?

In the mainstream school or the unit provision, the question changes to:

• How much time will Jamie spend with a qualified teacher of the deaf?
• How will that time be used?
• How much training will be given to mainstream and support staff?
• How will the teacher of the deaf and the mainstream teachers work together?

Curricular issues

Simply being part of a mainstream school that offers a broad and balanced curriculum does not ensure that Jamie will have access to it. To some extent, this will be strongly linked to the provision made to support his linguistic progress and his communicative needs, but it will also be linked to the subjects and skills of the teaching staff, their own practical teaching style and their willingness to differentiate the curriculum for him and any other children with special educational needs. Jamie's special educational needs will sometimes be better catered for by the support assistant or teacher of the deaf withdrawing him either individually or with a small group. If he is withdrawn, however, it is important that he still covers the same subjects and aspects of curriculum that his hearing peers do, although some of the emphases may differ. For this reason, there will need to be very careful joint planning by the mainstream teacher, the teacher of the deaf and the support staff so that Jamie's right to a broad and balanced curriculum is not compromised. Not all teachers in mainstream classes make their planning available in this way, although the increasing use of 'service level' agreements, in which services and schools draw up a contract detailing roles and responsibilities for meeting a child's special educational needs – what each will do and provide, what the aims of the provision are and so on – has considerably facilitated this.

In the mainstream and specialist unit provision, the curriculum on offer to the deaf child should look very similar to that available to other pupils, and the challenge for the school and specialist support staff will be to maximize the deaf child's access to that curriculum while catering for the child's special educational needs. In the specialist school, the meeting of the child's special educational needs should not be an issue if the child's placement is appropriate; the challenge will be to deliver a curriculum that is as extensive as that in mainstream schools and that supports children to high levels of attainment.

Although non-maintained and independent special schools do not have to deliver the full National Curriculum, most deaf children have Statements of SEN that require them to have access to a broad, balanced and relevant curriculum, including the National Curriculum. Attending the specialist school is part of the provision for that access rather than an indication that a different curriculum is necessary. If a school has a roll of fewer than 60, there may be many advantages in terms of its intimacy, its ability to support children's personal social and emotional well-being, its general ethos and its tailoring of individual programmes to meet need. If it is an all-age school, however, it may struggle to provide specialist subject teaching in all subject areas, and standards within those subjects and the qualifications taken and gained by children may suffer as a result. Many schools for the deaf have small numbers and yet cater for a wide age range; a single class may include children from differing year groups and with a range of curricular and special educational needs needs. It is important that parents have a clear idea of the make-up of the proposed class for their child and how such differing needs will be provided for. Deaf children in mainstream classes may also not have full access to some subjects or to standards equivalent to those of others if curricular decisions taken for them are influenced by when staff support is available and what curricular areas specialist staff feel they can adequately support.

Jamie's parents will want to know:

- Is the full National Curriculum delivered?
- What range of qualifications do the children, including those with hearing loss, take at the end of their schooling?
- What levels of attainment do the deaf (and hearing) children reach in National Curriculum core subjects (English, maths and science) in the national tests at the end of each key stage (at ages 7, 11 and 14)?
- How does this compare with children's levels when they entered the school?

Learning and support issues

Much provision for deaf children recognizes the necessity for the learning environment to be at times very deliberately tailored to meet their special educational needs through, for example, individual and small-group learning opportunities with support and teaching staff. In the mainstream, the extent of this provision will be linked to the child's current level of linguistic functioning, listening and attending skills, the demands of the curriculum and the particular classroom or school organization.

Most severely and profoundly deaf children will, however, need some such provision daily if their language and listening skills are to improve. To this end, the support provided is used in a variety of ways – class support, withdrawal and small-group work with other deaf/hearing children. Some parents and mainstream teachers have strong views about the amount of support that should be provided for children, some in fact feeling that the child should have support for almost the whole of the school day. The advisability of such provision is, however, much in dispute. Deaf pupils themselves appear to find such intensive support intrusive (Bown, 1997) and detrimental to their self-confidence. It may inhibit rather than facilitate their relationships with mainstream teachers and interfere in their friendships with other pupils.

Those working with all children with special educational needs are now recognizing that there is a fine line between support and dependency. A high level of individual support and small classes may be extremely advantageous for deaf children; however, too much attention can be as restrictive to children's learning as too little. In particular, there is a danger of fostering what Fraser (1990) terms 'learned helplessness' as children demonstrate dependence on adults and a lack of confidence in their own ability to learn without support. Taking responsibility for one's own learning and thinking for oneself are important parts of children's personal and intellectual growth. Jamies's parents will want to ask:

- How does the school provide for this?
- Are there enough opportunities for individual and small-group work?
- Is there too much adult supervision and support?
- Do the sorts of activity they are involved in challenge children to think for themselves?
- Are children allowed to make mistakes and learn from them?

Technical and audiological support issues

Deaf children have very specific technological needs, and it is important that wherever they go to school, equipment is used optimally and audiological needs are monitored, evaluated and met. All approaches to the education of deaf children recognize the importance of maximizing the use of residual hearing through effective and appropriate hearing aid provision and use. At preschool level, parents and teachers of the deaf work together with the hospital audiological services to ensure that children are wearing working hearing aids all the time. Daily hearing aid checking routines will be firmly established in the home, alongside regular electroacoustic testing, in Jamie's case once a week. Jamie's parents have a small range of spares at home and emergency telephone numbers ensuring that Jamie never has to be without two working hearing aids for more than 24 hours.

When he goes to school, Jamie will continue to need such high-quality amplification provision and support. Most schools for the deaf have high levels of on-site audiological provision and at least one teacher of the deaf who has additional qualifications and responsibility for audiology.

Children at mainstream schools and specialist units will need the same level of technical and audiological support made available to them. There will need to be clear procedures in place for checking Jamie's aids, organizing spares and notifying the teacher of the deaf of any problems. Someone within the school will need specific training for this, but all staff in contact with the child will need a basic level of training in using the child's amplification equipment appropriately and checking its functioning.

Although parents, and the children themselves, will take some responsibility for the equipment, research shows that this is not enough, even with apparently competent listeners. Smith (1994) provides evidence that the day-to-day audiological management of children is variable once they reach compulsory school age, whatever type of school they attend. In Smith's study, around 60% of children's hearing aids, taken directly from children's ears, were not working optimally, often because of minor faults. In addition, many were being worn at inappropriate volume and gain settings. There were significant differences, however, in the number of faults found in hearing aids worn by children in total communication specialist school settings and in those worn by children in the auditory-oral school for the deaf or mainstream settings. A significantly higher proportion of pupils in auditory-oral contexts were wearing appropriately functioning aids and using the gain of those aids more effectively. Smith's sample of specialist total communication – and indeed auditory-oral – provision was small, and it may be that others have more (or less) effective checking routines, but the warning is there for all. Simply having the audiological facilities does not guarantee that children are wearing working hearing aids appropriately set. Hearing aids can go wrong at any point during the day, and some children's effective access to the curriculum will stand or fall on the technical support and provision that is made to support them. Jamie's parents will ask:

- What audiological facilities and equipment will be provided?
- Who will carry out electroacoustic testing?

- How often?
- How will aids be checked on a daily basis?
- When will Jamie use an auditory trainer/FM system?
- What happens if an aid is not working?
- Will Jamie have access to an educational audiologist?
- How are hearing aid settings evaluated?
- What training will be given to the mainstream staff?

Personal and social issues

The advantages of local mainstream provision for supporting deaf children's inclusion into family and community life have already been considered. However, simply being in such provision does not ensure that such benefits are reaped, and some deaf children, despite 'coping' with the academic elements of mainstream life, do not find within the mainstream school the support they need for personal well-being and social and emotional growth.

Recent research (Harrison et al., 1991) demonstrates the majority of deaf children to be well placed in such contexts and to have the same friendship and emotional maturity ranges as their hearing peers. Other research, however, shows the picture to be more variable (Lynas, 1986; Gregory et al., 1995) and underlines the importance of reviewing the provision for all aspects of the deaf child's needs, including social and emotional ones. One child may be at ease, achieving and feeling valued within one school community. A different child with a different personality and strengths and weaknesses may be visibly stressed and/or socially isolated within the same context. For such a child, irrespective of level of academic attainment, alternative support patterns and/or a more specialist placement may have to be considered.

Some parents feel very strongly that their child will be more comfortable in an environment that includes other hearing aid wearers and that has been established solely with a view to meeting their needs – a specialist unit or school for the deaf. Indeed, for some parents and children, it is a relief to meet other hearing aid wearers and an adult community totally at ease with hearing loss. Most deaf children come from hearing families, however, and not all settle readily into the predominantly deaf community with which they are confronted in specialist schools. Not all parents, on visiting a school for the deaf, feel that their children will be comfortable in its ethos, and many are anxious about how their child will develop the skills to fit into the wider community of hearing people. If children board, there may be the problem of keeping up local friendships and of the child's involvement in home and community life. Parents will need to plan more carefully to support their child's needs for satisfying social relationships with both deaf and hearing peers. One of the benefits of specialist units for the deaf children is that the child has available a potential peer group of other hearing aid wearers, some of whom may have difficulties similar to those of the child concerned within the context of a more mainstream environment.

Most schools will have a personal, social and emotional development policy designed to support the deaf child's increasing independence, awareness of others, initiative, moral values and self-esteem. Parents will need to feel comfortable with the values and beliefs that the school promotes and the emphases that it places. The questions to consider are:

- What opportunities are there for children to take decisions and to take responsibility for their own learning and actions?
- Are deaf children given responsibilities in school similar to those that hearing children will have?
- Does the school have a behaviour policy?
- How will matters like sex education and spiritual awareness be dealt with?

Partnership with parents

All schools have statutory responsibilities that they must fulfil in terms of reporting to parents about their children's progress and involving the parents of children with special educational needs in annual review procedures and target-setting for the child. Parents will have played the pivotal role in their child's life and early education, working closely with their visiting teacher of the deaf, taking their child to clinics and to nurseries and having daily contacts with teachers there. Specialist units and schools for the deaf are rarely within walking distance of children's homes. Even when the children are day pupils, only a small percentage of parents take their child personally to a school for the deaf, and a similarly high proportion of children who attend resource bases are 'taxied' by the LEA to school. Where the deaf child attends the local school, contacts between teachers and parents will be frequent, and involvement in school activities as accessible as it is to all other parents. If the specialist unit or school for the deaf is not nearby, such contacts may become more formal and infrequent; parents may not be able to visit the school very often and may feel increasingly excluded from their children's experiences.

Most schools and units recognize these difficulties and work hard to keep parents as involved as possible. Many use home–school notebooks to give daily or weekly information about school events, work covered and interesting things the child has said or done. Regular school bulletins and details of topics that children will cover are sent home, so that parents can share their child's interests and learning. In residential schools, text-phones, amplified telephones, e-mail and fax facilities enable parents to keep in regular contact with children and staff. For all provisions, parents' meetings and other school events, including workshops on key aspects of children's learning, all help parents to feel part of the school community. Some residential schools have family accommodation to enable parents to attend such workshops, make more extensive observations of their child in the school and attend their child's annual review.

All schools will have a 'partnership with parents' policy. Jamie's parents will wish to read this and will also want to talk with other parents about how this operates in practice:

- How are parents kept involved in their child's education and broader school life?
- How will the school involve them in target-setting for Jamie and in evaluating his progress?

Residential issues

There are obvious questions that parents will want to ask about the after-school care that children receive in residential schools. Most can only be answered by visits and observations when the children are in residence. Very few schools now have large dormitories, preferring children to be in smaller 'family groups', each with its own care staff. Some parents have mixed feelings about the close relationships that their children establish with these other carers, as Amy's mother indicates:

> Whenever she comes home, she is full of what she's done with J. I'm really pleased that she's happy, but she seems to do so much and sometimes I feel that I can't compete. We have so little time at weekends before it's time to go back, and by the time we've gone shopping and washed her clothes.... I try to do something every weekend but that's not always possible. I've talked to J. about it and she says that Amy spends most of Monday and Tuesday talking about us, so perhaps I am overreacting.

A range of extracurricular activities may be organized for children to join in with, some school based and some within the local community. Homework will be supervised, and children will have some free time to simply relax or occupy themselves. They will increasingly be expected to make decisions about the activities and interests they wish to follow.

It is sometimes very difficult, however, for residential schools to strike an effective balance between the need to offer careful supervision for other people's children and the children's needs for privacy, independence and to learn to organize and prioritize. Although most residential environments in schools for the deaf are very effective, a small number have been accused of being too prescriptive and overprotective. There is a danger that, in such circumstances, children will not develop the independence and self-help skills that they will need in the broader community once they leave school.

Rights and responsibilities: the law in the UK with regard to children with special educational needs

Under current legislation and guidance in the UK, LEAs have a qualified duty to provide for pupils with special educational needs in mainstream schools, providing that the provision is appropriate for the child's identified needs and that such a placement is compatible with the efficient education of other children and the efficient use of resources.

The law on special education is contained in the 1993 Education Act. The Code of Practice (DfEE, 1994) provides guidance to schools, LEAs, health authorities and social services in the form of a framework for meeting special educational needs. It outlines a five-stage model that seeks to involve parents at every stage and within which schools and LEAs have differing responsibilities according to the stage on the model or register of special educational needs at which the child is placed. The model represents a continuum of need from stages 1 and 2, where, in general, the responsibility for drawing up an IEP and setting out targets rests entirely on the school, to stage 5, at which the LEA considers the need for a Statement of SEN, draws one up if appropriate and arranges, monitors and reviews provision for the child (DfEE, 1997).

Providing for the needs of children under 5

At this point in Jamie's life, his parents are unclear on what his specific needs on school entry and beyond might be and how and where best to provide for them. They and Jamie do, however, have a number of rights even before he reaches 2 years of age, and there are certainly current special educational needs that must be provided for if Jamie's later educational pathway is to be smoothed.

The Code of Practice (DfEE, 1994) considers that Statements of SEN will only rarely be necessary for children under 2 years of age, although parents have the right to ask for a statutory assessment if they have grounds for concern at this stage. LEAs are, however, encouraged to establish appropriate individual programmes for babies and children with special educational needs, within both homes and development centres. The Code recognizes that children will have special educational needs before compulsory school age and encourages all preschool providers to be proactive in identifying and providing for pupils' special educational needs.

Certainly, Jamie and his family already receive a range of LEA services, including twice-weekly visits from his teacher of the deaf, attendance at a specialist parent toddler group, ongoing hearing aid evaluation, technical support, toy library facilities, regular reviews and video analysis of Jamie's progress. This provision is based on an initial assessment of need by the audiological and education personnel, followed by 6-monthly reviews of progress towards the objectives set for Jamie. A statutory assessment of Jamie's needs will be made closer to school entry, unless Jamie's parents feel otherwise.

Provision for school-age children

Each school has responsibilities to identify and assess children's special educational needs. Any special provision made for children who are placed at stages 1 and 2 on the school's Register of SEN will come entirely from the school's own budgets. Such children will have an IEP setting out detailed targets and programmes for them and success criteria against which progress will be judged. Children who are placed at Stage 3 on the school's Register of SEN are pupils for whom the school needs to call on the expertise and support of external specialists.

Many hearing aid wearers will automatically be placed at stage 3 by schools in recognition of the ongoing need for support, advice and sometimes direct teaching from peripatetic teachers of the deaf that the child might require. At stage 3, both external specialists and schools have certain duties and responsibilities. The overall responsibility for meeting the child's needs is still retained by the school, but external specialists must provide advice to the school about teaching styles, programmes and activities, and may contribute to both the teaching and assessment process. In reality, the amount of time and resource that peripatetic teachers can commit to stage 3 children will depend on the LEA's special educational needs support and funding policies. Such policies – and the amount of money for special educational needs provision that LEAs have delegated to schools – vary considerably. Schools in one LEA will pay for or 'buy in' teacher of the deaf services for stage 3 children, whereas in another they will not. Such distinctions alone have resulted in children with very similar needs being placed on different stages of the Code – one at stage 3, another at stage 5, for example – because they live in different LEAs.

Statutory assessments and Statements of SEN

Stages 4 and 5 are the stages for which the LEA takes clear responsibility for defining and assessing children's needs and considers whether a Statement of SEN is appropriate. At stage 4 following referral the LEA considers the need for a statutory multi-disciplinary assessment of the child's needs and carries out the assessment if it is determined appropriate. There are very clear guidelines given to authorities on procedures to follow at stages 4 and 5, personnel to be involved, time limits that must be met and information that must be given to parents while the need for an assessment and subsequently a Statement of SEN is being considered and the Statement itself prepared. It is at stage 5 that the LEA considers the need for a Statement of SEN, prepares the Statement, makes arrangements for provision and monitors and reviews the provision's effectiveness in ensuing years.

This chapter is not the place to pursue a detailed exposition of the statementing or annual review process. Many very effective guides have already been written for parents, and the LEA itself must supply parents with written information of the process, their rights and the name of the 'Named Person', independent of the LEA, who can help to guide parents through the process. Such Named Persons are often connected with voluntary agencies who specialize in supporting the families of children with special educational needs, but parents can also identify their own alternative Named Person whom they wish to support them.

The National Deaf Children's Society advises and supports parents, suggests Named Persons and has produced a range of booklets to help parents through the statementing process. Other useful sources include the Advisory Centre for Education's 'Special Education Handbook' (1996) and the Independent Panel for Special Education Advice, who will provide free assessments, help and advice.

Statements of SEN

The final Statement has 6 main parts:

Part 1: Personal details.

Part 2: Summarizes the child's special educational needs, strengths and weaknesses. This should reflect the assessments that have been carried out and the advice submitted by both professionals and parents, including, in the case of a deaf child, advice from or written following consultation with a qualified teacher of the deaf. If there are conflicts in the evidence received, the LEA must resolve this and indicate why it has occurred.

Part 3: Details the special educational and developmental objectives that are to be achieved through the Statement and all the special educational provision that the LEA considers necessary for the needs identified in Part 2 to be met. The provision must be 'specific, detailed and quantified'.

   Arrangements for monitoring the child's progress, for the annual review and for setting shorter-term targets will also be specified.

Part 4: Names the school that the LEA has decided is appropriate and will be left blank in earlier drafts of the proposed Statement until parents have had opportunity to express their preference for a particular school.

Part 5: Details non-educational needs such as occupational therapy, physiotherapy and speech and language therapy

Part 6: Details the provision that will be made to meet these non-educational needs

Before the final Statement is issued, parents will be given a copy of the proposed Statement and all the evidence and advice given. They then have 15 days in which to respond, either by making representations to the LEA, meeting with an officer of the LEA and/or expressing a preference for a particular school.

The majority of parents of children with special educational needs, including deaf children, accept the analysis of needs and the provision made, and agree with the suggested placement. It is in fact often the placement they suggested. In such circumstances, a system of annual reviews swings into place once the final Statement has been issued. At each annual review, the child's progress is considered and the following questions asked:

- Have the child's needs changed?
- Is the provision still appropriate?
- Is progress sufficient?
- Does the Statement need amending?

Parents have opportunities to contribute their own reports and their views on whether the school is still providing for their child's statemented needs. If they have any doubts, they can ask for a reassessment of special educational needs.

Parents' rights to contribute to the assessment process and to challenge LEA decisions

The vast majority of Statements of SEN are drawn up, agreed and delivered in schools without any real dissent between the LEA and parents. In a small number of cases, however, this is not so. To understand how such dissent might arise, it is important to understand the various procedures that support the statementing process, the components of a Statement and the rights that parents have within this.

In the Code of Practice (DfEE, 1994), there are many recommendations made about the involvement of parents at stages 1, 2 and 3, but it is only at stages 4 and 5 that parents have actual rights in law. Parents have, for example, the right to request a statutory assessment and, unlike other referral agencies, can demand a response from the LEA within 6 weeks of making the request (Gravel, 1997). LEAs must investigate the nature of the concern even if they ultimately decide not to make a statutory assessment. Once the referral for statutory assessment has been made, parents have three major ways of influencing the process and the decisions that are made.

First, they can exercise their right to submit detailed evidence on their child's needs and the appropriate provision that should be made for them.

Second, parents can make representations to the LEA at each stage of the process and can submit evidence from their own independent advisers. Parental evidence will also include their views on the type of help the child will need in school – the provision to be made. In this case, provision does not mean which school but rather the resources, the help, the teaching styles and the programmes that will support the child's learning. Earlier in this chapter, we explored some of the needs that might be identified and the provision that might be made: audiological provision, support from a qualified teachers of the deaf and/or from trained support assistants, provision for curricular access, training for mainstream teachers and so on.

Parental evidence should be in as much detail as possible at this early stage and should centre on their child's strengths and weaknesses, his needs, his experiences to date, the provision they would like to be made and their hopes for the future.

Third, parents can exercise their right to discuss the proposed Statement at a meeting with an officer of the LEA, where they can explain their views, present their evidence and suggest alternative wording for the parts of the Statement they wish to see amended. Such suggestions may or may not be agreed by the officer but can be resubmitted in writing by parents within 15 days of the final meeting. At such meetings, LEAs are not allowed to cite their own guidelines as explanations for proposed provisions. Parts 2 and 3 of the Statement must be a consideration of the child's needs and effective provision for them rather than of the child's needs in the context of LEA resources and existing provision. Only when the final Statement is issued and the placement is decided can 'the efficient use of resource' be taken into account, and then only if the proposed placement can meet the child's needs. Parents have a right to express a preference for a school in the maintained or non-maintained sectors, but LEAs have only a qualified responsibility to comply. If they do not accept the parents' preference, they must indicate why that school is inappropriate.

A recent SEN Tribunal case contested just such an issue when Jonathon, a Year 6 child, was due to transfer to secondary school. Although he had received an auditory-oral education to date, the LEA proposed a transfer to a specialist resource for hearing impaired children where total communication was used and much of the in-class support was from communicators who used sign with the deaf pupils. Jonathon's parents requested a reassessment and, while this was being carried out, visited a number of alternative secondary schools, including one maintained by a neighbouring authority that had a number of deaf pupils on roll and was visited regularly by a teacher of the deaf. This, they indicated, would be their preferred placement. The final Statement named the LEA's own school and resource base so the parents appealed, not simply against Part 4 of the Statement, but also against the LEA's description of Jonathon's needs in Part 2 and the provision to be made in Part 3. Their case centred on the fact that Jonathon did not now need a total communication approach (this being confirmed by an independent report from an educational psychologist) so that placement at a school where the main approach used was total communication was inappropriate. The LEA evidence for Part 2, however, included the need for Jonathon, for personal, social and academic reasons, to be in an environment in which signs were used. At the Tribunal hearing, the LEA, having conceded the parents' and their expert's evidence on the inappropriateness of total communication for Jonathon, still considered that his needs could be met within the named specialist resource base. It could provide no clear reason, however, why he should not attend the school of his parents' preference and was ordered by the tribunal to name that school as the appropriate placement in Jonathon's Statement.

Once a child has been referred for statutory assessment, there are three points at which parents have rights of appeal to a SEN Tribunal:

- if the LEA decides not to carry out a statutory assessment
- if the LEA decides not to issue a Statement of SEN
- if the parents disagree with Part 2, 3 or 4 of the final Statement, i.e. against the description of the child's needs, against the description of special educational needs provision that is specified, or against the school that is named or if no school is named.

In addition, parents can appeal:

- if the LEA refuses to comply with a request to change the school named or decides to cease to maintain a Statement.

The SEN Tribunal was set up to provide an independent and legally binding resolution when parents disagreed with the LEA. The LEA itself must provide parents with information about the SEN Tribunal and their right to appeal, and there are very definite procedures and time limits to be adhered to when appealing to and presenting evidence to it. Despite the view of many professionals that the system is too parent-friendly (Thistleton, 1997), many parents report feeling overwhelmed by the volume of paperwork, the need to understand what is legally arguable and the presentation of the case to the hearing itself. In 1995, there were 1551 appeals registered to the Tribunal across the range of special educational needs. Of these, 48% were withdrawn. Some of these withdrawals were undoubtedly positive as parents and the LEA came to a compromise acceptable to both. Others, however, represent parents who felt worn down by the process, as Gravell (1997) recounts:

> One mother I know was called into school for three hour long sessions with the head, who tried everything he could to get her to withdraw her appeal, even though the dispute was about speech therapy provision and not to do with the shortcomings of the school. She did withdraw, because she didn't want her son to suffer from any effects of the dispute on the school's relationship with her ... Her son's therapy has been withdrawn recently due to a funding crisis in the local NHS Trust and she has no legal recourse.

The SEN Tribunal will hear evidence from the LEA, parents and witnesses, and make a judgement on whether the LEA has reached the right decision for the child in the particular circumstances specified in the Act. Wherever possible, it will try to get LEAs and parents to agree rather than simply impose such a judgement.

Most appeals are completed within 5 months, and parents and their witnesses can claim travel expenses and subsistence. Nonetheless, the appeals procedure is costly in time, energy and resources, and the Green Paper 'Excellence for All' (DfEE, 1997) suggests that LEAs may in future be required to offer parents a conciliation meeting at key decision points when areas of disagreement and possible options will be considered. Such meetings might involve a person playing a neutral role, such as one of the Parent Partnership Officers already working within some LEAs.

As someone who at times advises parents on how to secure resources or a particular placement decision for their child, I have often seen the breakdown in communication that can occur between parents and schools or services once parents have indicated that they do not necessarily agree with the LEA's assessment and certainly not with parts of the proposed Statement of SEN. Any moves that support more effective discussions between parents and the LEA can only be to the benefit of deaf children, whose parents, teachers and LEA are often diverting huge resources of time, money and energy into the preparation of appeals, resources and time that could be much more effective if they were diverted into children's programmes.

We need furthermore to restate that the vast majority of deaf children's parents and their LEAs are in agreement over the most effective provision to be made for them, and the mechanism for reviewing and evaluating their progress should ensure that this continues to be the case if the system is used effectively. Parents need to feel confident that the provision that is made for their deaf children can and does meet their special educational needs. Understanding their rights, the rights of their children and the duties of the LEA can only aid them in this and enable the 'partnership with parents' that is part of government, LEA and school ideology to become a reality at individual child level.

Summary

Concerns over the most effective school placement for their child are raised early by the families of deaf children, who need opportunities to gain information and to visit placements in their child's preschool years so that they can reflect carefully on which environment they feel will best meet their child's needs. This chapter has discussed some of the issues that parents and professionals must be aware of when exploring provision.

There are a number of general considerations that will be taken into account, but there will also be questions that are specific to a particular child. The more general considerations relate to communication issues, teaching and learning issues, curriculum delivery and access issues, technology issues and geographical issues. Since there are no 100% guarantees of success within any approach to the education of deaf children (see Chapter 5 for an overview of the current position), it is important that professionals recognize parents' right to inform themselves further, to choose not to follow advice, to look at alternative placements and approaches and to establish different priorities in relation to needs than those the professionals themselves might have.

The starting point for any discussions about schooling will, for most parents, be the teacher of the deaf, but some LEA services for deaf children, including Jamie's authority, also arrange a programme of talks and visits for parents. Local authority information packages give parents details of the provision made for children with special educational needs in that area. Other information packs clarify the statementing process and parental rights within this. Parents will want access to OFSTED school reports and the published GCSE and other results that demonstrate the attainments of deaf children at various stages of their educational career.

Deaf pupils go on to universities and colleges, to training schemes and directly into work; they become chefs and teachers, office workers, farm workers, lorry drivers, supermarket workers. In short, there are very few qualifications or employment opportunities that are unavailable to them because they are deaf. Like all children, the quality of education that they receive and the expectations that they and adults have will have an impact not simply on their academic qualifications, but also on their life opportunities when they leave school. Effective education for deaf children is about the right placement for each child. The legal framework underpinning special educational needs provision in the UK acknowledges and places certain responsibilities on LEAs to provide for this. It also allows parents (and children) certain rights to influence, if not always to determine, the process, including the right to challenge decisions and to present evidence to a Tribunal for SEN.

We have explored the range of placement options that are available for deaf children in the UK and some of the advantages and disadvantages of each. A major theme throughout has been that the right placement for a particular child, like Jamie, will be one that can meet all his special educational needs. It will be a placement in which he can learn and achieve, and not just cope, one which will indeed provide him with the skills to 'flourish in adult life'.

References

Advisory Centre for Education (1996) Special Education Handbook: The Law on Children with Special Educational Needs. London: ACE.

Bown M (1997) When should a school for the deaf be considered? Paper delivered at DELTA Professional Conference, November 1997.

British Association of Teachers of the Deaf (1995) The BATOD Survey (1994), Northern Ireland, Scotland, England, Wales. Journal of the British Association of Teachers of the Deaf 19(2, 3, 5); 20(2).

Deaf Education through Listening and Talking (1998) The Education of Deaf Pupils in Mixed Provision – A Policy Statement. DELTA (in preparation).

DES (Department of Education and Science) (1978) Special Educational Needs (Warnock Report). London: HMSO.

DfEE (Department for Education and Employment), and the Welsh Office (1994) Code of Practice on the Identification and Assessment of Special Educational Needs. London: HMSO.

DfEE (Department for Education and Employment) (1997) Excellence for all Children: Meeting Special Educational Needs. London: Stationery Office.

Fraser BC (1990) The needs of hearing impaired children and integration. In Evans P, Varma V (Eds) Special Education: Past, Present and Future. London: Falmer Press.

Fraser BC, McLoughlin MG, Pitchers B (1996) An Introduction to the History, Current Provision and Future of the Education of Deaf and Hearing Impaired Children. Available from Unit 2, EDSE 37, School of Education, University of Birmingham.

Gravel C (1997) SEN Tribunals: Weighing up the system. Special! Autumn 1997, pp. 13–15.

Gregory S, Bishop J, Sheldon L (1995) Deaf Young People and Their Families: Developing Understanding. Cambridge: Cambridge University Press.

Harrison DR, Simpson PA, Stuart A (1991) The social and emotional development of a population of hearing impaired children being educated in their local mainstream schools. Journal of the British Association of Teachers of the Deaf 15(5): 121–5.

Lynas W (1986) Integrating the Handicapped into Ordinary Schools – a Study of Hearing-impaired Pupils. London: Croom Helm.

Lynas W, Lewis S, Hopwood V (1997) Supporting the education of deaf children in mainstream schools. Journal of the British Association of Teachers of the Deaf 21(2): 41–5.

Powers S (1990) A survey of secondary units for hearing-impaired children, Parts 1 and 2. Journal of the British Association of Teachers of the Deaf 14(3): 69–79;

14(4): 114–25.

Powers S (1996) Deaf children's achievements in ordinary schools. Journal of the British Association of Teachers of the Deaf 20(4): 111–23.

Smith MS (1994) Children's Use of Hearing Aids. Unpublished PhD dissertation, University of Manchester.

Thistleton L (1997) SEN tribunals: an appealing procedure. Special! Autumn 1997 pp. 10–11 NASEN. Hobsons Publishing.

UNESCO (1994) The Salamanca Statement and Framework for Action on Special Needs Education. World Conference on Special Needs Education: Access and Quality, Salamanca, Spain, 7–10 June 1994.

United Nations (1994) The Standard Rules on the Equalisation of Opportunities for Persons with Disabilities. New York: UN Department of Public Information.

Winton PJ, Bailey DB (1994) Becoming family centered: strategies for self-examination. In Roush J, Matkin N (Eds) Infants and Toddlers with Hearing Loss. Baltimore: York Press.

All the Acts of Parliament cited in the text are published by HMSO.

Chapter 8
Learning to listen

JACQUELINE STOKES

For parents, the identification of a hearing impairment in their child may be a traumatic and bewildering experience. In addition to the emotional shock, many parents lack the information that will help them better understand and secure the support they need during the first months and years following identification. Many hearing professionals, however, tend to focus on the medical diagnosis of the hearing impairment and the technical solutions available. Based on the assumption that the solution to the problem of deafness resides in the proper use of the technology, they tend to emphasize the business of educating parents in how best to deal with the technology – hearing aids, radio systems, cochlear implants and so on – and overlook the way in which the introduction of the technical solution can impact on the communication and bonding between parent and child. This focus can mean that hearing specialists fail to understand, or be sensitive to, parents who are overwhelmed by the diagnosis.

Permanent childhood hearing impairment has many, far-reaching implications for the child and his family. Its effect on the development of spoken language is the particular focus of this chapter. It illustrates how parents and professionals can work together to enable the child to become a confident communicator.

This chapter is organized around a case study following the experiences of a child, Chloe, and her parents, from her birth through the first months and years of intervention and treatment for her hearing loss.

Chloe was chosen for two reasons. First, she is profoundly hearing impaired. This means that she was born with very, very little hearing. In general, it is true to say that the deafer you are, the harder it is to learn to talk, so the challenge for Chloe was great. Second, Chloe's hearing loss was identified very early. This meant that she had the advantage of being fitted with hearing aids at 3 months old, an advantage because many hearing impaired children are not identified until 18 months of age or even older. The case study details how Chloe made excellent use of the little hearing she has. The steps she took in learning to listen – her auditory development – are annotated in the chapter (AD1, AD2 and so on) and are listed together in the Appendix to this chapter. She showed us that, like normally hearing children, she communicated very effectively long before she began to use words. When words did begin to appear, they were used to achieve the same ends as in any normally hearing toddler. Chloe followed a very normal pattern of acquiring and using spoken language. The contributions from her parents, Ray and Sally, give insight into some of their particular concerns during Chloe's first 2 years.

While the case study is based primarily on one little girl – Chloe (whose case study appears in italics throughout) – the narrative also draws on the experiences of Monica and Georgia, and their parents. This gives a more comprehensive picture of the eventualities that can occur in the process of the identification of hearing loss and hearing aid use. Monica also has a profound hearing loss but, unlike Chloe, Monica's hearing loss was not identified early: she was 13 months old when the diagnosis was made. Georgia also has a profound hearing loss, which was identified at 3 months of age, and she demonstrates the advantages of being fitted with hearing aids at such an early age.

The chapter is written from my perspective as an early language adviser who has worked with families of hearing impaired children over many years. I work in an audiology department that has a long tradition of identifying hearing impairment early and providing good support for hearing aid users. I come from the auditory-verbal tradition, which seeks to enable the child to make the very best use of the hearing he has. In describing the process of identification and hearing aid use, this chapter draws on the basic ideas underpinning the early language programme offered to parents in our department. A central feature of the programme is the frequent video recording of interactions between mother and child, which illustrate the procedures employed to help the hearing-impaired child to learn to listen, to understand and to use spoken communication. The chapter includes excerpts from many hours of these video recordings.

1 January 1993

Chloe is born and is admitted to the special care baby unit because of a chest infection. Like all other babies on the special care baby unit, Chloe is routinely tested for hearing loss. The results indicate that she should have a further hearing test when she is a few weeks older.

6 February 1993

Chloe's parents return to hospital for further testing of Chloe's hearing. They have no concerns about her hearing. They report that she jumps

*when the dog barks and is making lots of baby cooing sounds. There is
no history of hearing loss in the family.*

*They watch as the audiologist holds a headphone to Chloe's ear and
can hear the very loud sounds going into her ear. Chloe does not stir.
Ray and Sally suspect that the audiologist does not know what he is
doing because the sounds do not even wake her up.*

*The audiologist looks in Chloe's ears and checks that the middle
ears, the parts of the ear beyond the eardrums, which house three small
bones, are working normally. Chloe wakes up and is not ready to co-
operate for any more testing.*

*The audiologist tells Ray and Sally that Chloe has a very severe
hearing loss. They are deeply shocked and saddened. They stay a while
and eventually leave with the news.*

*The audiologist organizes appointments with the ENT consultant
and with the early language adviser. Letters explaining the results go
immediately to the teaching and support services (visiting teachers of
the deaf), the GP and the health visitor for information and support.
Hearing aids are ordered, with a provisional plan to fit them when
Chloe is 3 months old.*

Breaking the news

Breaking bad news to a parent can be very difficult. Most people receive
no training in carrying out this difficult task, yet the professional's skill in
delivering bad news can have a profound effect on how well the family of
a hearing impaired child cope with the child's disability. It is important
to consider the way in which the news is communicated, for example the
native tongue, time allocated, verbal information, supporting written
information, the best environment in which to break the news – somewhere private and comfortable where there will be no interruptions –
and who should be involved and present. Parents need to be informed
of bad news clearly and tactfully, and at the earliest appropriate opportunity. Experience tells us that the process of giving information about the
diagnosis and the implications of hearing loss typically extends over
several months (Lincoln and Louth NHS Trust, 1996).

Telling parents that their child has a permanent hearing loss is particularly difficult when, like Ray and Sally, they have no concerns about
hearing. Some parents, however, have long suspected a problem and
relate the struggle that they have had trying to convince their GP, health
visitor and others to take their concerns seriously and do something about
it. Some of these parents experience relief on hearing the news – perhaps
it is better than their darkest fears – whilst others are deeply shocked, even
when they have been the ones fighting to get a hearing test.

Monica's mum, Val, had worried for many months. When Monica was
8 months old, a health visitor routinely tested her hearing using the
distraction test. (In this test, the child responds to noises made behind

him by turning towards the source of the sound.) Monica 'passed' this test, but Val continued to worry. The family eventually arrived at the audiology department when Monica was 13 months, and they learned that she was profoundly hearing impaired. This degree of deafness means that only the very loudest sounds, of pneumatic drills, lorries and low-flying planes for example, are heard.

Remembering the events 2 years later, Val said:

> So it was very obvious at that stage that something was really drastically wrong. I think it is awful really. I remember saying to John [the audiologist], when he said your child has definitely got a very severe hearing loss, he said you seem very shocked and I said, well I am shocked, I didn't think it was that bad. He said, but you're the one who told us she had a hearing problem so why has it shocked you? But I remember thinking, I was still convinced it was just a blockage in her ears. I had heard about children having grommets and I just said, ok what do you do now?
>
> Although I had suspected she had a hearing problem I didn't think it would be anything permanent. But then I said to him, what do we do now then? And he said, well we can't do anything about it other than give you hearing aids. And I said, what about grommets? He explained that Monica's problem was an inner ear problem and not a middle ear. I said, how do you know that? You haven't even looked in her ears! He said, if it was a middle ear problem then the hearing loss wouldn't be that great. And I said, well you must be able to do something. You can cure nearly everything these days. You must be able to do something. John said, No, no, can't do that. I remember saying what about if I sell my house and had lots of money. Could I pay somebody to put it right? But no that wouldn't do any good either. It is very hard to believe in this day and age that they couldn't do anything. I was convinced there must be some little operation, you know. I think I thought they'd say, yes, your child has got a bit of a hearing problem, bring her in next week and we'll sort it out and that'd be the end of it really.

February 1993

During February, Ray and Sally take Chloe to see the paediatrician in the baby clinic and the ENT consultant in the audiology department. At these appointments, tests are organized that might throw some light on the cause of the hearing loss. One of these tests is an eye examination. The ENT consultant checks Chloe's middle ears, nose and throat and finds them to be healthy and functioning well. He reviews the information collected so far and explains the results to Ray and Sally. He recommends that hearing aids should be fitted as soon as practicable.

Why your baby needs hearing aids now

Babies do a lot during their first year, including a lot of listening. Research shows that babies listen even before they are born, and at birth a baby already prefers to listen to his mother's voice (DeCasper and Fifer, 1980). Babies as young as 1 month can hear differences between speech sounds such as /pa/ and /ba/ (Aslin et al., 1983). During their first months, they learn to associate sounds with events and to tell an angry voice from a friendly voice. By 9–10 months old, they begin to understand commonly used words and phrases. By the time they are 1 year old, they have been listening for thousands of hours.

Children learn listening and language skills most efficiently in the first few years of life. During the early years, sound stimulates the growth of nerve connections between the infant's ear and the area of his brain that makes sense of the sound. Normally hearing babies are stimulated with sound all day, and this results in a rich network of connections between the ear and the brain. Depending on the extent of the loss, hearing impaired babies receive a significantly reduced amount of sound stimulation. Hearing aids increase the amount of sound reaching the inner ear and therefore stimulate the growth of auditory pathways to the brain. One or two hours a day of hearing aid use is not enough to provide the baby with the listening experience he needs to make sense of sound. Only full-time use provides the essential stimulation that his auditory system is missing. Broadly speaking, if the child only wears his aids for a quarter of the time he is awake, it will take him 4 years to get as much listening experience as a normally hearing infant has in 1 year.

February 1993

Chloe is 6 weeks old and is at the hospital for the first of many early language sessions. Ray and Sally describe Chloe as a very easygoing baby. She makes good eye contact while her parents play and chat with her. Chloe responds with lots of cooing. Both parents have a very natural interactive style with Chloe.

Ray and Sally are overwhelmed by the sadness they feel at the news of Chloe's profound hearing loss. Ray feels this particularly acutely when he is at work and unable to check that Chloe is all right. They feel unprepared because they know no-one with a hearing problem. Chloe's grandparents do not believe that Chloe is really deaf; they do not believe that it is possible to tell so early, as she is only 6 weeks old. Their feeling is that someone surely will be able to fix it.

Both parents put much store by the fact that Chloe's hearing loss has been detected early, which they believe gives her an enormous advantage. They also express great confidence in the reputation of the hospital.

What is early language intervention?

In the UK, over 90% of hearing impaired babies are born to hearing parents. Like all parents, they want to do the best they can for their child and are anxious to know what they can do to make it better. For most children with sensorineural hearing losses, caused by damage to the inner ear, there is no operation that will restore hearing. (In extreme cases, where the hearing loss is very severe to total, a cochlear implant may be an option (see Chapter 6). The loss is permanent and will have far-reaching effects on the child and his family. Many parents feel unprepared for their role as the parents of a hearing impaired child.

At this point, the family are introduced to a range of professionals who want to assess and evaluate their child, yet more who want to make suggestions and give advice, and others who are there to help. It is no surprise that some families complain of feeling overwhelmed. The success of early intervention depends crucially on how effectively professionals listen to parents. Giving advice and information is of little benefit if the parents are not emotionally ready to receive it. It is important that the many professionals who come into contact with the child take the time to explain their role to parents. There needs to be understanding about areas of responsibility and expertise so that parents are clear how each professional can contribute to their child's well-being (Watson and Lewis, 1997).

Teachers of the deaf typically offer advice and support to the families of hearing impaired children. In some regions of the country, this job may fall to, or be shared with, a speech therapist with specialist training in hearing impairment. In Reading, it is shared between the early language adviser and visiting teachers of the deaf. The main role of the early language adviser is to help to develop communication between the family and the child who does not hear well. This involves giving parents information to deal with hearing aids, as well as encouraging effective communication. Despite being aided, the child still does not hear perfectly and perhaps does not hear at all. An individual plan is drawn up in consultation with parents and other family members; this forms the basis of the early family support. The plan reflects parents' hopes and aspirations for their child and family, as well as their current concerns. The plan is reviewed several times a year in order to keep pace with changes in the child and the family.

The goal of early intervention is to strengthen parental confidence and skills as they learn about hearing impairment. Parents must be at the centre of each early language session and be given information, skills, techniques and access to resources in order to make informed choices about their child. It is important for them to learn why aids are needed, how to care for them and how to get them quickly into full-time use. They also need to understand the importance of play in language learning, to incorporate sound as something new and meaningful and fun in everything they do with their child and so on. All this information is needed – but not all at once.

Children normally learn language through being with caring adults who enjoy chatting and playing with them as they go about their daily routines. Hearing impaired children can learn language in the same way provided they are appropriately aided and hearing rich and meaningful language. The way in which parents talk to their babies is very special and helps them to learn language. Hearing impaired babies also need lots of this special talk. In each language session, emphasis is placed on looking at the ways in which parents talk to and play with their babies. Some parents of hearing impaired babies naturally use 'baby-talk'. Others find that communication becomes very strained and unrewarding for both parent and baby. This is for a myriad of reasons: the diagnosis of the hearing loss, the way in which the diagnosis was reached and given, the presence of the hearing aids and the strain of trying to talk to a child who does not hear well, together with strong and unexpected feelings of sorrow, regret or anger.

The overall aim of the early language sessions during the first 18 months is to give parents the skills and knowledge they need to be confident and effective in their role as parents of a child who, in addition to everything else, happens to have a permanent hearing loss.

April 1993

At 3 months old, Chloe is fitted with two powerful miniature postaural (behind-the-ear) hearing aids. The volume control is set at 2+. Child-proof battery locking compartments and volume control covers are fitted.

Impact of hearing aids on the family

The challenge of keeping hearing aids on an infant of whatever age should not be underestimated! In the early weeks, some parents find it an almost impossible task, whilst for others it is as easy as falling off a log. The age of the child seems to have nothing to do with it. It is no easier to keep aids on a 3-month-old baby than an 18-month-old toddler.

Sometimes there is a 'honeymoon period' when the child seems to take to the hearing aids and wears them happily. After a couple of weeks, however, when the novelty has worn off, the child wants nothing to do with the aids.

There is no simple solution to this. Each child reacts in his own special way. However, there is a fund of experience that resides with the teachers of the deaf, audiologists and other parents of hearing impaired children who have travelled the same road. There are many techniques that work for some children. Two of the most successful are distraction (putting the hearing aids on while the child is busy doing something else) and negotiation (capitalizing on a child's desire to do something – 'First we'll put your hearing aids in, then we'll feed the ducks'). The drive to find a technique that works depends on understanding the potential benefit of the hearing aids for your child. It takes time to see the benefit, and this leads to a 'Catch 22' situation: we need to see the benefit before we can muster the energy to win the battle, but the benefit cannot be seen until the battle is won and the aids are in frequent use. Keeping hearing aids on requires much more than mere perseverance, patience and creativity!

Monica's mum, Val, recalls how the hearing aids marked Monica out as different:

> I think getting the hearing aids was a bit of a shock because I knew she was deaf but I could hide it from other people. She was only a baby, so she didn't talk much anyway. But once she had the hearing aids in everyone could see them. I wasn't very keen on that to start with. You do get people looking and staring. I've got used to it now. I remember we were in the supermarket and Monica was in the trolley, and a lady went past like this [staring] and my sister said, 'What're you b... staring at? Haven't you seen hearing aids before? People staring at her, there's nothing wrong with her – she's only deaf, you know!'
>
> They did embarrass me too, I suppose. I think sometimes they still do. I wasn't ashamed of her or anything. It did embarrass me but I don't really know why. Probably just because you haven't got the ... In a way it's not as bad as losing a child, but in a way ... it's like, I didn't any longer have the Monica I thought I had. I had a different child then. It did embarrass me but I don't know why. I think it still embarrasses my mother and my sister because whenever my sister takes the children out, she tells me not to put her radio aid on because she doesn't want people to see it. It obviously still embarrasses her as well.

April 1993

Chloe is three and a half months old. After the first week of wearing the aids, Chloe's parents notice that, when Chloe is wearing hearing aids at home, she startles and becomes upset when the dog barks (AD1) (see Appendix p. 229).

Ray and Sally are happy to have Chloe videotaped wearing her hearing aids. The tape captures some of Chloe's vocalizing, which is loud, persistent, sounds like the vowel 'ah' and changes when she puts her fingers in her mouth.

Chloe appears to still in response to Sally's laugh. She is sitting on Sally's lap facing away, so the stilling may be in response to movement or sound or a combination. Chloe's vocalizations overlap with Sally's.

There is no smooth turn-taking yet, but Sally is trying to fit her talking into the spaces Chloe leaves in her vocalizing.

Chloe's head control is developing, so her aids are sitting well and there is little feedback (whistling coming from the hearing aid) in a supported sitting position on Sally's lap. Ray and Sally are having no trouble inserting the earmoulds. Feedback is a problem in the car seat and other places where the sound is cupped and gets channelled back into the aids. Impressions are taken for new earmoulds to be fitted in 1 week. Chloe is already able to dislodge and remove her aids.

Ray and Sally notice how visually alert Chloe is and talk about this as an advantage she has over hearing children.

Early communication

It used to be thought that babies did not do much during the first 12 months! Many people still think that communication begins when words emerge, usually between 12 and 18 months. However, if you listen to parents talking to babies, it is clear they are communicating:

Georgia: (rubbing eye)
Mother: Are you tired? Tired baby?
          (rubbing Georgia's back)
Georgia: (looks at Mum, small cry)
Mother: (turns baby so they are face to face) What? You're a
          real faker, you're a little faker.
          (broad smile)
          Yes you are. There's nothing wrong with you.
Georgia: (still looking at Mum)
Mother: No there's not.
          (moves baby so they are at the same eye level) There's
          nothing wrong with you. You're being silly.
          (broad smile)
Georgia: (small cry)
Mother: You're being silly. Yes.
Georgia: (looks down to side)

The important point here is that the mother acts as though Georgia is communicating. She responds with comments and questions to the baby's vocalizations, gestures, movements, coughs, smiles and burps. She pauses in between speaking and looks expectantly at Georgia, waiting for her to hold up her end of the conversation. She responds warmly to Georgia, smiles and uses a caring tone of voice. The conversation goes on until the baby looks away. In this way, the baby gradually comes to learn the basis of communication: that is, that one person says something, and the other waits, listens and then gets a turn to say something. This turn-taking is the basic structure of the way we converse. Georgia is learning how to communicate long before she understands or uses words.

Conversation between adult and child can be likened to a game of catch. Each person takes a turn to throw the ball, while the other gets ready to catch it and then throw it back. The ball is the topic of the conversation, and the game clearly works best when both partners are throwing the same ball back and forth. In conversations with babies, the topic is chosen by the adult and is often to do with the baby: what he's doing, where he's looking and so on. In this way, the parent begins the important process of telling the baby about the things he is interested in. Such joint attention is vital to the development of communication.

Chloe's case history details her progress through the prelinguistic stages (communication using everything except words) to the emergence of symbolic language (using spoken words or signs). Like many hearing impaired babies who are identified early, she followed the normal pattern observed in hearing children and at broadly the same age.

April 1993

After 2 weeks with the aids, new moulds are fitted. Chloe is very talkative and enjoys vocal play with her mum and dad (AD3). Ray and Sally observe that Chloe is noisier when she wears her aids (AD4).

Anne, her childminder, has noticed how Chloe whinges when she leaves the room, and this makes her come back in. Chloe has discovered that her voice is an 'attention-getter' that works.

Gaze patterns

What is it about babies that gets us hooked? It is something in the eyes. When a baby responds by making eye contact and we can sustain the gaze long enough to get a smile, this is reward enough for talking to the baby. The crucial role of eye contact in early communication is brought home in an fascinating study of blind infants by Fraiberg (1979). A blind baby who smiles 'looks happy' and one who is crying 'looks unhappy', but it is difficult to read other feelings in between these two states. A blind baby does not 'look quizzical', 'look interested' or 'look doubtful'. He has a very limited number of facial expressions. Fraiberg reports how her team came to read the blind baby's feelings from watching his hands.

When watching videotapes of parents talking to their young babies, it is intriguing to see how the baby's mood is mirrored in the parent's face, smiling when baby smiles, sober when baby is distressed, laughing sympathetically when baby looks indignant. These signals provide the most elementary and vital sense of communication long before words have any meaning.

Together with orienting movement, gaze is the first means by which we can detect what infants are paying attention to. Parents respond by following the infant's gaze and talking about it. The child eventually comes to understand more of what is said because it is about something to which he is already paying attention.

May 1993

Three weeks after hearing aids were fitted, the first attempt at measuring Chloe's response to sound is tried in the audiology room. Wearing her hearing aids, Chloe stops moving and stops vocalizing in response to loud warble tones. The tones are loud – 80 dBSPL – and deep pitched. High-pitched sounds are tried, but Chloe's response is less obvious for these. This is an encouraging first testing session.

Early responses to sound

Just what kind of response to sound do we expect following hearing aid fitting? Up to about 6 months old, children do not usually turn when they hear a sound. The only clue they may give to having heard is a slight stilling or eye-widening. Even when the infant is older than 6 months, he may not respond to sounds until he has started to learn to listen.

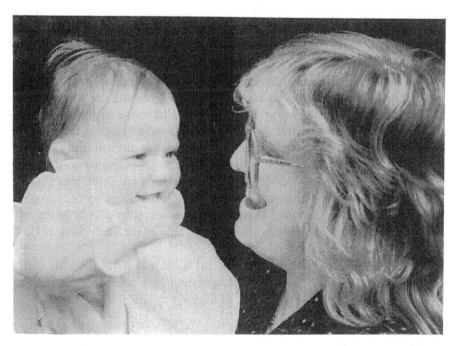

Figure 8.1 Baby Chloe makes eye contact with her Mother, Sally. Only 4 months old and so much to say!

Hearing aids are designed to enable the child to detect speech sounds. Unfortunately, they also amplify all the other sounds in the world. Gradually, the child learns the difference between one sound and another, and in time is able to sort the important sounds from the background noise and select what he listens to.

This sorting of the wood from the trees is what learning to listen is all about. It is a long process and does not simply happen. For some profoundly deaf children, it may take many months before any benefit from hearing aids is really clear. The length of time it takes does not always relate to the degree of hearing loss represented on the audiogram. Experienced teachers of the deaf know that children with similar audiograms can have vastly different listening abilities. Dr Ling, a pioneer in the world of deafness, likens the audiogram to a shoreline: it tells you where the water is, but it does not tell you how warm it is. In other words, it tells you how loud the sound must be for the ear to detect it, but it does not tell you about the quality of the message sent to the brain.

Chloe clearly demonstrated a benefit from her aids. When her aids were put on in the morning, her voice went on too. Her parents said, 'She likes the sound of her own voice. For however long she has the aids on, she just goes on and on and on until she just conks out!' (AD4). However, her parents were able to cut into Chloe's monologue by making eye contact and talking to her. This showed that Chloe had the ability to quieten herself in order to pay attention to her parents. It was an indication of her potential to learn to listen (AD2).

At the time of hearing aid fitting, parents are often asked to look for signs of loudness discomfort. This is an extremely difficult thing to be asked to do. How can you decide whether the child is upset by the loud sound or the movement that accompanies it? Does she cry when I shout at the dog because my voice is too loud or because of my cross face? Some months after a fitting, a mother mentioned in passing that her son still cried when his sister played her recorder. She did not think that this was evidence of loudness discomfort but more his response to what was then a truly unmusical noise! Can a 3-month old baby tell you that his aids are too loud? He may not be able to link his upset to the aids, but babies are very effective in letting us know when they do not like something! Most children remove their hearing aids in the early days. Is this a sign of loudness discomfort?

Children are inquisitive beings and have a natural interest in the things in their ears. One mother explained just how vigilant she was having to be during the first week of hearing aid use by her 4-month-old baby. She said:

More than likely you turn your back for five minutes and she's got them in her hand. 'Did you want these Mum?'

And what power! Pull out your hearing aids and poof! Mum appears within seconds.

Some children constantly remove just one hearing aid. This is more often a sign of their being right- or left-handed rather than of one aid being too loud. Many children, like Chloe, do not enjoy wearing aids in the car. In Chloe's case, this was probably due to the amount of engine noise interfering with how well she could hear herself!

May 1993

Chloe is 4 months old and has now had her aids for a month. Mum and Dad are both back in full-time work. Sally brings Chloe to the first appointment of the day each week, then drives to the childminder, then into work. Ray brings Chloe when his shift allows.

Chloe is awake a lot now during the day, taking cat naps, and is eating a variety of prepared baby foods. She uses her hearing aids for most of the time she is awake and is becoming more aware of the sounds around her.

Directing attention/sharing attention

During the early months of life, the baby gradually becomes interested in objects as well as people. These objects become the topic of parent–infant chats. Here, Sally explains how, when Chloe was 5 months, she was able to direct her attention in play with a pop-up toy:

> Mickey's in the middle and Goofy's on the end and Donald Duck's on the other end and they make noises. And we say 'Which one's Goofy?' and I think she's getting to know which one's which. And I say 'Get Goofy, get that one (point), get Goofy' and her hand will go up to it.

Sally uses gaze, gesture and voice to direct Chloe's attention. Now both are looking at the same thing. Mum names the object of their shared attention, and, over time, through this much-practised routine, Chloe begins to understand more and more of the verbal part of the message. Chloe's mum recognizes this as a new development, and it is – Chloe is showing that she can pay attention to something of her mother's choosing. A lot of time is spent following the infant's lead in play and conversation, and it is equally important that the child comes to follow his parents' lead.

June 1993

Chloe is 5 months old and has had aids for 2 months. The new earmoulds allow the aids to be turned up to volume 3 without feedback occurring. Chloe is quite dextrous and can take off her aids very swiftly. Sally wants to try 'Huggies' to help the aids stay in place, although this will not help her to put the aids on a wriggling Chloe. (Huggies are small, flexible plastic rings that loop around the hearing aid and the child's ear. They are designed to stop the aid from flopping off the ear.) She is also trying an elasticated headband that goes over the ears, being careful not to obstruct the microphone.

Chloe's eye sight has recently been tested and found to be ophthalmologically satisfactory.

Chloe is videotaped again this session. The contrast between her vocalizing when she is aided and unaided is striking. Chloe is clearly louder and more vocal with her aids on. Sally responds by becoming louder and more animated. When wearing one aid, Chloe stills and slowly turns in response to a loud feedback from her other aid.

Chloe has started to giggle, causing delight all round. She cries when Mum shouts at the dog (AD5). We use the videotape of Chloe to review our planning for the next few months.

Use of videotape

Videotaping is an essential tool for charting progress during the early years, and many teachers and speech therapists use it for just that reason. In the early language programme, videotape plays a central role. Each child is videotaped for 10 minutes, at least monthly in the early stages. This is partly to chart progress. It is also the only way to capture and replay the fleeting events so characteristic of interactions with infants. Did he look at the ducks when you said 'Quack quack' because he heard and understood you, or did you glance at them first and give him a clue? It also allows the rest of the family to see at least part of the weekly session at another time and in another place.

Videotape is particularly useful for looking at parents and infants interacting together. The main purpose is to observe various aspects of their interaction to see where their strengths lie. Sometimes it is useful to use a checklist, such as the one by Cole (1992), to record the key points.

Videotape is a useful tool to spot how the adult naturally promotes listening. A short segment of the infant and parent together is sufficient to see how the adult notices sounds, how face and body language is used to alert the child to listen, how the parent observes the infant's reaction to sounds and how the parent responds to the infant's reaction to sounds. Of course, parents are also the source of the sounds they want their child to listen to. One mother complained, 'I was told to just keep talking to him and he would learn to listen but he doesn't pay any attention to me.' She did indeed need to keep talking to him, but in that special way that adults do to little children, called 'baby-talk' or 'motherese'. It is a style of speech almost always used by adults when talking to infants and is distinct from the way of talking to adults and children who are no longer babies. Some aspects are easy to spot: the exaggerated intonation patterns, the lengthy pauses left for the baby to respond, the prolonged eye contact, the repetition of key words and phrases, the facial expressions and gestures. Babies seem programmed to attend to 'motherese'.

The videotape is best studied by the language adviser or teacher of the deaf and the parent together. It is important to be aware of cultural differences in the way in which parents play with and talk to their children. In some cultures, parents do not believe that they should follow the child's lead or expand the child's utterances (Crago and Eriks-Brophy, 1993). A sensitivity to these cultural issues would seem to be a prerequisite to any parent guidance. Typically, parents are very self-critical and rarely need anyone to point out just what they are doing wrong. It is rather more useful to look at what they do that is helpful to their child's play and language development. These joint sessions generate plans for future play and language opportunities.

July 1993

Chloe is now 6 months old. The session is videotaped. Chloe is able to sit unsupported for 10 minutes at least. She is becoming much more interested in toys, and everything goes in her mouth. She can pay attention to either toys or people. The tape shows that she is singularly interested in a plastic ring that she is holding, mouthing and eventually drops. Sally offers to retrieve the ring and does so. All the while, Chloe looks at the ring. She is not ready to share attention between Sally and the toy. We can anticipate that, over the next few months, Chloe will signal to Mum that she wants her to retrieve the ring by looking between the ring and Mum.

A new sound is appearing in Chloe's repertoire: 'mmmm'. This is heard when Chloe is feeling cranky and when she is mouthing toys.

To make 'mmmm', all you have to do is continue to vocalize with your mouth shut!

August 1993

At the age of 7 months, Chloe is showing that she is beginning to turn to sounds around the home so is ready to try some aided testing using visual reinforcement audiometry (VRA). On this occasion, she responds to warble tones by stilling and making very clear, slow turns towards the speaker and the visual reinforcer. The sounds are loud (65–75 dBSPL), about as loud as a shout from a few feet away, and are in the low and middle frequencies (0.5 and 1.0 kHz). This is a short session as Chloe quickly tires.

Frequency of support

The amount of support that hearing impaired children receive varies widely across the country, from one 'advisory' visit per month, to several per week. Children on the early language programme at the Royal Berkshire hospital are seen weekly in the audiology department by the early language adviser and at least weekly at home by the visiting teacher of the deaf.

Each weekly session at the audiology department lasts an hour. During this time, problems with earmoulds, tubing, battery supply and hearing aid faults are dealt with, and impressions for new moulds and the fitting of moulds takes place. Very young babies who are growing rapidly require new earmoulds regularly, particularly when the loss is severe and extremely well-fitting moulds are required. This may mean that up to two sets of new moulds are fitted each month. It is also an opportunity to check the child's hearing responses with and without aids and to monitor the state of the middle ear. A few minutes spent testing frequently is more efficient than trying to do a lot in an hour-long hearing aid review appointment every 3 months or so.

All this effort is in recognition of the very real difficulty of trying to keep hearing aids on a young infant. The presumed benefit of early detection and fitting of hearing aids drives the move towards universal screening for hearing loss in babies. Fairly obviously, the benefit only accrues when the aids and all that goes with them outweigh the imposition experienced by the family.

August 1993

Chloe is still 7 months old and has been aided for 4 months. Another session is videotaped. Chloe's vocalizing is changing and sounding like the vocal play stage heard in normally hearing babies between 4 and 7 months of age. There is a greater variety of vowel-like sounds, she is experimenting with intonation, 'mmmm' is frequently heard in long tuneful sequences, she plays with the extremes of pitch, and long pitch glides and raspberries punctuate her chatter. She is now having two long naps a day, worn out by all her talking.

Chloe's awareness of sound is carefully observed. On this occasion, she shows the first signs of recognizing a sound – a whistle – by looking at its referent, a bird mobile (AD2). The sound of the bird whistle had been linked with a bird mobile on many, many occasions before.

Making listening meaningful and fun

Hearing impaired children become motivated to listen as they discover that sound has meaning. The full force of this statement is caught in this early experience of a deaf person who never benefited from hearing aids. She writes of one early childhood memory:

> I watched my mother as she opened the door to our apartment and greeted a visitor. Several times I watched. Every time she opened that door someone was on the doorstep. Great! I loved visitors. So I tried. No one was there. I shut the door, puzzled. Later I tried again. Still no one there. Then, without warning, my mother would suddenly walk to the same door and open it. Always, someone was there. I was truly vexed. Did Mother have magic powers to make visitors appear? (Tucker, 1995)

Parents are encouraged to draw their child's attention to sounds around the house so that the child becomes aware of them and gradually associates them with the source. The objective is for the child to learn what makes each noise so that he can eventually tune them out and concentrate on the important sounds of speech. No-one wants to spend his days jumping up and pointing to his ear every time an aeroplane flies over.

The child becomes motivated to listen through meaningful and fun interaction with parents.

October 1993

After 5 months of hearing aid use, with Chloe now aged 9 months, her parents report on her listening skills. They notice that, at meal times, Chloe follows their conversation across the table by looking from one speaker to the other, in the manner of the umpire at Wimbledon! (AD8). She also turns around when called and when Mr Ben, the dog, barks.

This opportunity is taken to continue evaluating Chloe's hearing aid benefit. On this occasion, she is wearing her aids at volume 2+. She responds to warble tones that are at 60–65 dBSPL by turning to the speaker and the visual reinforcer. She responds to all the pitches tested: the deep pitches, the middle pitches and the high pitches. She also responds to voice at 50 dBA. This confirms the observations that have been made of Chloe's growing ability to detect voice and sounds around the house.

What does she actually hear?

At a hearing aid review appointment, the audiologist takes time to talk to parents about their child. He listens to their concerns and asks questions about the child's progress. Together, the audiologist and the parents plan how best to use the allotted appointment time. The audiologist normally explains the tests beforehand and discusses the results afterwards. This is an opportunity for parents to ask the audiologist questions and try to discover the relationship between the test results and what their child can actually hear in the real world (see Chapter 3).

At the first hearing aid review, it is useful to begin measuring what the child can hear when wearing his hearing aids. To do this, sounds are made through a loudspeaker, and observations of the child's responses to these are made by the audiologist. The audiologist tries to find the quietest sound to which the child responds. This is measured in decibels (dB). The audiologist repeats this procedure using some low-pitched and some high-pitched sounds. The frequency of the sounds is measured in hertz (Hz).

Even when the intricacies of how hearing is measured and what the hearing aids do are understood, it is still hard for parents to understand what their child really hears. This is because the answer depends on a range of factors.

Let us take Chloe as an example. First of all, the results from the hearing aid review showed that Chloe stopped her play when she heard sounds that had an intensity of 60–65 dBSPL. This is about as loud as a strong voice close by. So when Chloe is kept close to the person speaking, she can hear that he is talking. This is useful information, but it still does not tell us what she hears. Does the word 'cat' sound like 'cat' to her?

Simply put, speech is made up of vowels and consonants. The vowels (a, e, i, o and u) tend to be low-frequency sounds, whilst consonants such as s, t, k and f are high-frequency sounds. So if a child can only detect low-frequency sounds, he will only hear the 'a' in 'cat'. Chloe can hear both low- and high-frequency sounds, so you might expect her to hear all of 'cat'. But there are more things to consider. High-frequency sounds such as s, h and f are quieter than the vowel sounds in normal speech. Thus the child needs to have better hearing in the high frequencies than in the low frequencies to hear all of 'cat'. Chloe hears the 'a', but the 'c' and 't' very faintly, if at all. Shouting 'cat' does not have the effect of making the 'c' and 't' any easier to detect. It simply makes the 'a' louder and drowns out the 'c' and 't'. Chloe has more chance of hearing the whole word if it is whispered very close to her hearing aids. This technique is called acoustic highlighting and is one of many tips for helping children learn to listen that are found in Ling (1989) and Estabrooks (1994).

This is still only part of the answer. The hearing test is carried out in a quiet, soundproofed room so that there are no competing sounds. (Actually, in our experience, most of our children are chatterboxes and provide plenty of competing sounds!) It is much more difficult to hear in a noisy environment, and the real world is of course full of background noise. So from this test alone, it is not possible to say what a child can hear in the real world. Parents are advised to be aware of background noise at home and to reduce it as much as possible.

A hearing impaired child has a much better chance of hearing when his parents speak close to the hearing aids. This works because sounds get louder as we get nearer to the sound source. A useful way to demonstrate this is with a tape recorder. The microphone of the tape recorder is essentially similar to the one in the hearing aid. Speak into the microphone at a distance of 6 inches, 1 foot, 2 feet, 4 feet and 8 feet, and keep your voice level the same. Shout at 16 feet; then go back to the microphone at 3 inches and whisper. Play the tape back and hear how dramatically your voice fades as you move away and how quiet the shout is compared with the whisper at 3 inches. The message is to move in closer to the hearing impaired child before speaking.

October 1993

Chloe is just over 9 months old. She is sitting in a seat that clips on to the table for today's videotaping.

It is becoming easier to attract Chloe's attention using voice alone. She turns to 'Chloe' or 'Listen', and she readily looks at whatever the adult is pointing out. Then she reaches for it and tells us she wants it, while looking directly at it. She is not quite ready yet to look between the toy and the adult to tell us that she wants us to give it to her. When she gets the toy, she explores it. Chloe pushes Sally's hand away when she does not want to give it up. She is learning to assert herself. Chloe is not only aware of voice, but also beginning to associate sound with action/object. On this occasion, Sally watches her looking at a toy aeroplane and makes the sound she has been associating with a flying aeroplane 'ahhh'. Without looking up, Chloe makes the aeroplane fly while Mum makes the sound (AD13).

Chloe continues to use her voice a lot. She is just beginning to imitate sounds in vocal play with her mum. She copies an 'ah' and 'uu', and makes different sounds when playing with train ('choo choo') and the aeroplane ('ahhh') (AD12). Extremes of pitch and loudness, squeals and shouting punctuate her playful voicing. There is a marked difference to be heard when she is trying to imitate a sound and when she is voicing to accompany her play.

Chloe is enjoying table-top play. She is learning the routine of first shaking the toy container to hear whether there is something inside it. Her full attention is taken by hide-and-seek games with a puppet, and she is discovering that her voice can make things happen, in this case make the puppet reappear. This is just one more step towards discovering that sound is meaningful and fun.

Play with stacking rings turns into a vocalizing turn-taking game. Chloe watches as we hold a ring up to our mouths, make a sound and pass it to the next person. She picks up a ring and offers it to her Mum and watches as she vocalizes. Chloe catches on very quickly.

Development of babble

Cooing is the first stage of babble, which all babies, deaf or not, seem to make between the ages of 2 and 3 months. The second stage is sometimes called vocal play or expansion. During this period, usually around the age of 4–7 months, the infant enjoys playing with his voice. His experiments with pitch sound like squealing, experiments with vocal quality sound like growling, and experiments with intensity range account for the yelling and whispering. He also seems to gain some control over his mouth and tongue, and, apart from the delight caused by blowing raspberries, he also tries deliberately to copy the mouth patterns of the adult by opening and closing his mouth and poking out his tongue. His sounds are more vowel-like, he takes part in back and forth vocal play when his sounds are copied, and his turns at talking are becoming smooth, with very little overlapping of speakers.

The next stage of vocal development is reduplicated or canonical babble. This is the 'mamama' and 'dadada' sequences that occur between 7 and 10 months of age. These strings of consonant and vowel rarely, if ever, occur in the vocalizing of severe and profoundly deaf children who have not been able to hear their own voices (Oller and Eilers, 1988). However, following hearing aid fitting, many of these children do develop reduplicated babble.

Between 11 and 12 months old, the child sounds as though he is talking – but in a different language. The strings of sounds have changed from the simple repetition of the same sound, for example 'mumumum' (reduplicated babble), to a mixture of vowels and consonants such as 'damibeba' (now called variegated babble). The first words usually appear between 12 and 18 months of age.

October 1993

Chloe is seen in the baby clinic at the hospital to discuss the results of tests to investigate possible causes of her hearing loss. The results of the TORCH test, screening for evidence of toxoplasmosis, rubella, cytomegalovirus and herpes virus infection, are negative. This means that some possible causes for Chloe's hearing loss have been eliminated. A referral is made for genetic counselling.

Chloe is now crawling, pulling herself up to stand and watching everything very closely.

Aetiology

Throughout the first few months following the diagnosis of a hearing loss, effort is made to determine the cause. For many parents, this is a crucial question to have answered, although frequently no cause can be found (see Chapter 2). Five years after the diagnosis of Chloe's hearing loss, Sally put it this way:

> Even now, five years on, it can still choke you up. You always ask yourself 'Why?' Because there's no ... it couldn't be explained. You know she had the tests that there are, into rubella and that sort of thing, but they all came back negative. It was one of those things that happened and that was it, and I suppose you sort of think why couldn't she have been like any other, but saying that she doesn't do too bad.

People deal with the diagnosis of a hearing loss in many ways. 'Getting to grips with it', 'getting on with it' and 'realizing what it means' is a process that can be long and overwhelming. Some parents tell later of thoughts they had which they shared with no-one at the time: 'I didn't want him to be deaf because it just isn't fashionable to be deaf.' Most professionals working with the family during this time recognize that the parents can be going through emotional turmoil and experiencing new and overwhelming feelings, but in our effort to do our job, we sometimes overlook this. We ask lots of questions, such as 'Does he respond to this sound?', 'Can he do this or that?', 'Do loud sounds upset him?' and 'How long does he wear his aids for?' The danger is that this can make otherwise perfectly sensible caring parents feel stupid and unobservant as they find they do not know the answer to these questions.

This is one of those situations where, if you have not had a deaf child, you simply do not know what it feels like. We can, however, learn from the parents of deaf children. One parent wrote that having a deaf baby was rather like planning a trip to Italy. She'd read the guidebook, bought the clothes and then got off the plane to find she had landed in Holland. It was the wrong place – she did not want to be there. But if she had spent her life mourning the fact she had never gone to Italy, she might never have discovered the wonderful things about Holland (Kingsley, 1991).

November 1993

At 10 months of age, a session is videotaped and used to look at the many ways in which Sally is developing Chloe's motivation to listen.

Sally lets me know Chloe has her first word: 'Did you tell Jacqueline you've been saying nana?'

Chloe has discovered her pointing finger. She is not yet using it to direct others' attention but will soon discover how useful it is in getting others to name objects for her, retrieve objects and so on.

Sally and Ray anticipate many of Chloe's needs and are trying to hold back a little to give Chloe an opportunity to tell them what she wants. She is on the verge of discovering that she can regulate other people's behaviour through her voice and a combination of eye gaze, pointing and reaching.

She waves bye-bye (AD13).

Development of pointing

There is more to pointing than meets the eye! Some ways of pointing are easier for the infant to follow than others. An infant of 9 months follows a point away from him, but he has to be about 14 months before he can follow a point across his face.

November 1993

Chloe is 11 months old. Her vocalizing is changing and now sounds like the babble of hearing babies: long strings of reduplicated babble – dada, baba, nana, mama, tete. She tries to imitate meow. Sally says that Chloe has been picking up rings and making sounds into them at home. This is caught on today's videotape.

Chloe enjoys looking at picture books and is beginning to point to the picture when asked to find 'the meow' or 'the woof woof' (AD12). 'Give mummy a kiss' (AD17) gets an appropriate response too.

Sometimes Chloe tells us what she wants us to do by looking at the object and vocalizing, and then looking at the adult. She has discovered how intentionally to regulate other people's actions. This coincides with 'out of sight' no longer being 'out of mind'. Lots of things are being dropped and then retrieved by designated adults!

Chloe loves table-top play and wants to get in the high chair as soon as she arrives. The bottle has been replaced by a trainer cup. This baby is growing up.

Adult-directed table-top play

The purpose of adult-directed play is to supplement the listening and communication that is part of everyday play and routines at home. During table-top play, the child's attention can become very focused on the activity when all competing noise and movement is kept to a minimum. The advantage of 'adult-directed' play is that all the elements needed for successful learning can be put in place. First, the child is motivated because the adult has chosen a toy that is novel and not available for play at other times, for example a jigger trigger, a stacking toy that pops the rings off when the trigger is pressed. Second, the child is able to do the game: it is neither too easy nor too difficult. Third, the child has a natural curiosity and is eager to see the rings fly up in the air. And fourth, the child is reinforced not only by praise, but also by the completion of the activity itself. The adult knows that the level of play is right when the child wants to do it over and over again.

Table-top play is an opportunity for Chloe to discover that her voice can make things happen; for example, calling 'baa' makes the lamb puppet appear, 'go' makes a variety of wind-up toys whizz across the table, and any vocalization makes the bubble wand appear. Emerging vocal play is reinforced by taking turns to copy sounds using the rings on a pop-up toy. The very routine of table-top play is helpful to the child: listen, the toy is presented in an interesting way, talk about the toy, use the voice to make it do something, play and talk about the toy, respond to the child's interest and communication, put it on one side, repeat the procedure and put the toys away. So much of the routine is familiar that the child can concentrate on the part which remains to be accomplished.

The disadvantage of adult-directed play is that it may be too controlling. The adult may override the child's communicative contributions in the effort to reach her own goal. It is possible that the watching parents may feel that this is how they should be playing with their child at home.

It is useful for everyone to take the time to observe the child while he communicates in good acoustic conditions in order to see the advantage of repetition, routines and so on. However, the goal of early language intervention is to make communication successful in the real world where there is background noise and other interruptions. All the time spent saying 'aaaah' and moving a toy plane around in the air is worth it when the child spots a plane in the sky and tells you 'aaaah'.

December 1993

Chloe is coming up to her first birthday and her first Christmas. On this month's videotape, Chloe shows us that her babbling has changed again and now sounds as if she is talking – but in a different language. Some single words are recognizable and used without prompting. Chloe says 'bye bye', 'grandad', 'hello' (on the telephone) and 'nana'. Along with the evolving talk are definite signs of early understanding. When asked to pick out 'the meow' from a small group of toys, she looks at the cat and sometimes picks it up.

Many of Chloe's turns now involve showing and requesting. She has learnt how to direct an adult's attention to something across the room by looking back and forth between the object and adult and vocalizing. On tape, she does this nine times in 2 minutes. The sound that accompanies her pointing sounds like the 'u' in cup. Videotaping this sequence shows which features of Sally's talk are responsible for keeping the conversation going around Chloe's pointing.

Chloe spends a lot of time singing to herself while gently rocking. She rocks while listening to music on the cassette player too (AD11). She enjoys singing with her parents, readily joins in (AD18) and asks for her favourite – 'Round and Round the Garden' – by pointing to her open palm.

She listens attentively for 20 minutes of table-top play. Chloe imitates actions and voice readily. She is a keen communicator who not only likes to talk, but is also ready to wait and listen, and to respond to her conversational partner.

Sally and Ray say that she tolerated her aids at their very noisy family get-together. They have also noticed that, although they think she understands 'No', she often does not stop when told 'No'!

Disability living allowance

This is a benefit for which families of all children with hearing impairment can apply. It is a tax-free Social Security benefit that is not means tested. A leaflet explaining the allowance and how to obtain a claim pack is available from post offices. The claim pack contains forms and explanatory notes. The forms are long and require considerable stamina. Teachers of the deaf and health visitors will often help to complete these forms. The National Deaf Children's Society provides a very helpful guide called 'Disability Living Allowance for Deaf Children and Young People'.

March 1994

Chloe is 14 months and has found a new way to get our attention – shouting! She is showing that she is making more and more connections between sound and objects. She looks around the room and locates the object when asked to find the 'quack quacks', teddy bears and whistling birds (AD19).

Some of her babble is strings of vowels and consonants. She has added 'tedted' (teddy bear), 'eye', 'there' and 'that' to her vocabulary.

Chloe is beginning to play with a doll, cuddling it and feeding it with a spoon (sometimes not very accurately).

Sally says that they are still getting lots of information and advice from friends on how to fix hearing losses. She finds this very tiring.

Play

Play is an excellent opportunity for adults to provide the rich language environment that their child needs to develop his early communication.

Children spend most of their day at play, and many parents try to find times during the day that they can devote to playing with their child. Unfortunately, these golden opportunities can turn into frustrating episodes for both parent and child when we turn play into work.

So what is play? Descriptions of play usually include the following features. First, it is fun. This does not mean that everyone has to be laughing and smiling but that players enjoy the activity and show this by repeating the activity over and over. The repetitive nature of play is sometimes irritating to the adult who wants to stop or change the activity long before the child has finished with it! Second, play serves no outside goals. The enjoyment comes from the doing rather than the end result. The infant who has just learned how to release things from his hand enjoys dropping things over the side of his pram and watching them fall. The willing adult who retrieves them and eventually says 'Now hold on to it' has a different idea about play. Third, play is voluntary. It is something children choose to do.

Unfortunately, playing with a child sometimes turns into a struggle of wills. Or perhaps the child simply gets up and plays alone somewhere else. This is occasionally because the child wants some time to play quietly on his own; often it is because adults and children do not play in the same way. Adults sometimes want to teach the child how to play with toys properly, and the fun goes out of it. Videotaping can help to analyse just what is going on when children reject our attempts to play with them. Adults who find it easy to play alongside a child tend to be responsive to his interest in the toys; respond even when he is communicating in non-verbal ways, for example pointing or making a facial expression; sit where it is easy for him to hear and to make eye contact; go at his speed; and let him know how much they enjoy watching all the clever things he does when playing.

April 1994

Chloe has been listening for 1 year. Her responses are measured using VRA. The aids are at volume 3.

The results are as follows:

Frequencies tested:	0.5	1	2	3	kHz
Intensity levels:	45	55	60	60	dBSPL

These are the best aided responses so far. Chloe's hearing loss at different frequencies can be estimated using information about the hearing aids. The results are of estimated headphone thresholds of between 80 and 110 dBHL.

Unfortunately, Chloe does not like the visual reinforcers used in the test room.

Chloe is regularly using a small number of words frequently and without prompting. They are: 'nana', 'mum', 'dada', 'hello', 'round and round', 'mu', 'baa', 'quack', 'meow' and 'woof'. She can pick out pictures of birdies, teddy, ducks, 'roar' (tiger), shoes and fish when Sally asks her to find them.

Why so much emphasis on audition so early? Why listen?

The primary reason for emphasizing audition (listening) is its key role in developing spoken communication. This argument is spelled out in Chapter 5. However, there are at least three additional reasons for developing the child's auditory sense.

First, there is the safety reason. A child who is aware of sounds around him may be alerted to the sounds of danger – the ice cracking, the fire alarm ringing. Sounds call our attention to events in the environment: the ice cream van coming, the doorbell ringing. In practice, however, the profoundly deaf child is much more likely to rely on his acute sense of vision for warning. He will certainly spot the ice cream van as soon as it turns the corner, long before he hears the jingle. Relying on the eyes to receive communication (whether sign or lip-reading) has safety implications simply because when the eyes are concentrating on signs or lips, they cannot be watching what else is going on around.

Second, an awareness of sound gives information about our place in space. Sounds become quieter as we move away from the source; having two ears allows us to locate the source of sound. Thus sound can give us information about where things are, how far away they are and from which direction they are coming.

Third, sound helps us to understand cause and effect. The knock on the door means that someone is there, the sound of dropped keys alerts us to their whereabouts, the engine noise lets us know that the car is running, and the sound of running water reminds us to turn off the taps before it is too late.

Sound is so integral to a hearing person's life that it is easily underestimated and undervalued. Children who learn to use their hearing as the means of learning spoken language have an advantage over those who are dependent on lip-reading: they can communicate in the dark.

May 1994

Sixteen months old, and Chloe is recognizing and understanding more and more of the little phrases used regularly in her daily routine. She understands 'Give it to mummy' (AD13) and 'Do you want to sit in the chair?' (AD17) when there are no visual clues given, such as pointing or glancing towards Mummy or the chair. Chloe overhears a discussion

*between her parents about 'round and round', promptly picks up a cog,
makes it go round and says 'round'.*

Chloe has added /k/ to her babble.

*At this stage, Ray and Sally feel that it would be useful to record
Chloe's use and understanding of spoken language. Both parents agree
to record when Chloe uses a new word spontaneously and frequently.
They also try to record which words she seems to understand in context
but unsupported by visual clues such as pointing.*

Receptive language

Receptive language comprises the symbols, words or signs that a
person understands. Children who are born with a hearing impairment or who acquire it before they are 3 years old are 'prelingually
deaf'. These children have to develop language while hearing only part
of the speech message. Even with hearing aids, Chloe is still unable to
perceive some of the sounds of speech. In noisy situations, the difficulty is even greater. Hearing impaired children such as Chloe learn to
understand spoken language through their eyes and their ears.
Initially, the association Chloe made between the whistle and the bird
mobile depended on the sound of the whistle, the pursed lips and,
perhaps, the feel of the breath stream. Gradually, the sound of the
whistle alone meant 'bird'.

Situational understanding is sometimes mistaken for receptive
language. Situational understanding develops from the predictability of
daily routines. Children link actions and events long before they understand the meaning of the words used. Compliance with 'Put your coat
on, it's time to go' will be due to Mum looking for her bag and standing
up long before any word is understood. In the early stages, it is difficult
to separate situational understanding and receptive language.

Understanding comes before use. The hearing impaired child does
not use expressive language until he has receptive language. A normally
hearing child spends much of his first year listening and developing
receptive language before the first words begin to be used. Typically,
receptive language grows at double the rate of expressive language: he
knows more than he says!

July 1994

*Chloe is 19 months, and the 'terrible twos' have arrived early: she is
throwing tantrums at the drop of a hat! Tantrums are at the top of
Sally's current concerns, and we build ways in which to manage them
into our individual plan.*

*Sally has noticed that Chloe is beginning to pick up a few simple
verbs now – 'blow', 'open'.*

Chloe has always been very vocal. Now she is using a lot of jargon full of almost comprehensible phrases. She makes herself understood by using the occcasional recognizable word amongst the jargon and also through her tone of voice, intonation, natural gesture and facial expression.

Chloe readily involves willing adults in her pretend play with dolls and tea sets. She is very visually alert and readily copies new ideas into her play.

Tantrums

Children do not always wait until they are 2 to begin the 'terrible twos' – 18 months is a popular starting point. There are many parenting books available to help us through this stage of child development so there is no need to take space here. However, two simple pieces of advice have been found to be very useful. First, do not ask a yes/no question if you are not offering a choice. Do not say 'Do you want your hearing aids on now?' unless you are perfectly content for the child to say 'No'. Second, on the topic of tantrums, think of the child as a sailing boat and the parent or adult as the wind. Take the wind out of the sails, by leaving the room for example, and the tantrum tends to stall. Read books like these, find something that works for you, and rest assured in the knowledge that every other parent of a child this age knows what you are going through.

August 1994

Chloe is 20 months old and very determined. Her total dislike of the visual reinforcers in the audiology test room has meant that we have to get ready for 'performance testing'. We are concentrating some effort on teaching Chloe to wait and listen for a sound. She shows us that she hears the sound by putting a man in a boat or a ball on a stick. Sally has become creative in the use of toys to keep Chloe interested in this task. Popping tiny plastic teddies into a bottle of coloured water is a favourite and provides another language learning opportunity (AD21).

Chloe is showing that she can understand and co-operate with simple instructions such as 'Teddy wants to go up up up the slide', 'Put teddy in the car' and 'Teddy's tired, he wants to go night night.'

Parent record: Chloe now uses 27 words and 7 animal sounds.

Another first, Chloe blew her own bubbles!

She is ready to play lotto and post the cards to put them away.

Hearing tests

Some 3 years later, Sally remembers all of this with alarming clarity:

The hearing aid reviews with the clowns were a nightmare. She hated the clowns and the dogs with the flashing lights. The puppet would come up and she went ballistic, and after that she wouldn't do anything. After that she wouldn't even go in the room until they had taken them out.

The first ones [hearing tests] were sort of vague really because we didn't know what it was all about. We didn't know what it meant. I don't think you are given enough explanation and even now I think, what does that mean then? Even now it is difficult. Even now I would love to be in her head and hear what she hears. At first it was all gobbledegook and it wasn't until they did tests without her hearing aids that we started to understand what she heard without them, which is 110 to 120 dB, which is very very deaf.

Chloe ably demonstrated what she thought of the hearing test. She voted with her feet: she simply refused to walk into the audiology room until the toys were removed. We moved quickly on to performance testing.

Performance testing relies on co-operation from the child. The child waits for a sound and, on hearing it, puts a ball on a stick or a man in a boat. This type of testing often begins between 2 and 3 years of age (see Chapter 1). Some children enjoy hearing tests; some do not. In real life, the hearing impaired child uses all sorts of clues to make sense of what is going on around him. He uses his vision, context, situational clues and speech reading, as well as his hearing. In the test situation, he has to rely on hearing alone – the one sense that is impaired – and this is difficult for him. It is hardly surprising to find that some children fidget, fail to concentrate or become distracted in an effort to get out of an uncomfortable situation.

October 1994

Chloe is 1 year and 9 months old. The game to encourage imitation that began with the rings many months ago is working really well. Now Chloe readily imitates: when asked, when she meets a new word and when her parents put particular stress on a word and leave a meaningful pause.

Chloe enjoys books and points and names familiar objects without prompting.

Chloe and her parents are deep in tantrum territory.

Another first: Sally reports that Chloe said 'Bye-bye daddy.'

Parent record: 50 words used expressively.

Expressive language

Expressive language is the use of symbols, signs or words to communicate ideas, feelings and needs. A child is using expressive language when he can use a word meaningfully and spontaneously, i.e. without being prompted.

The sounds the hearing child makes gradually change from cooing to reduplicated babble to canonical (or varigated) babble to first words over the first year. The child's communication gradually becomes more intentional as he learns to convey his wants and needs through the co-ordination of voice, eye gaze and gesture. Children are competent communicators long before the emergence of symbolic expressive language. Imitation plays a role, as we have seen with Chloe. Babies first imitate themselves, seemingly endlessly throughout the first months of hearing aid use. Then they learn to copy the sounds that parents make in play with toys. Gradually, they begin to copy words when asked and even when unprompted. A period of 'jargoning', follows when the child is practising talking but no-one is really sure what he is trying to say! It is clear from the description of Chloe's expressive language that she has broadly followed this normal pattern of language development.

November 1994

Chloe is 22 months old. This session is videotaped to look at the language that Ray and Sally use when talking to Chloe. Chloe's language is changing daily. By looking closely at the video, it is possible to see how refinements can be made to make her language environment even richer and more tailored to her language level.

Rich language

As children become better communicators, the language that adults use also changes. In the early months, parents respond to cries, burps, and even sucking, by asking questions, commenting as they take care of the baby. This quite quickly changes, and parents become more selective about which sounds they will respond to. This usually coincides with the 'expansion' stage of babbling in which many more 'speech-like' sounds begin to emerge.

The nature of the adult's response also changes as the child begins to use words. Parents engage in modelling and expansion. Modelling is giving the child the words he needs to express himself right now. To be successful at this, the parents have to quickly assess the situation and read the child's mind. Expansion describes the kind of response that builds on the child's utterance. The expansion can be of different kinds. For example, a child points at a life-size poster of a tiger and says 'Roar'. One expansion might be 'Roar, that tiger roars.' This is a grammatical expansion. Another type of expansion builds on the meaning 'Roar, oh I'm frightened of the tiger, roar.'

Expansion is one way of making the child's language environment richer. Expansions frequently occur in normal parent-to-infant talk (Cross, 1977) and are thought to be helpful to young children learning language. This may be because children more readily imitate adult utterances that are expansions.

Chloe's videotape showed that Ray and Sally's efforts to get Chloe to take part in conversations with them were paying off. As a baby, they responded to her every move in an effort to help her to keep up her end of the conversation. At that stage, Chloe understood none of what was said to her. Now the situation has changed, Chloe is understanding simple language, and her parents are having to think about ways of enriching the language they use with her.

December 1994

Chloe is almost 2. In this session, Ray and Chloe are videotaped. The success of Ray and Sally's efforts to make sound meaningful for Chloe is amply demonstrated on today's tape. Play with puppets, including a snake who hisses 'sssssss', is later followed by a listening game. Chloe waits, listens to a sound – 'a', 'u', 'i', 'sh' or 's' – and responds by putting a stacking soldier together. On first hearing the 's', Chloe immediately goes in search of the snake, finds it and comes back to the job in hand. Chloe not only listens, but also connects the sound with an object.

She responds to loud or new sounds by pointing to her ear and saying 'What's that?'

Chloe is using many single words to do a lot of things. Her latest additions are: 'Uh oh' (I dropped it), 'Want that', 'stop it' and 'Chloe'.

Ling six sound test

The six sounds 'm', 'a', 'u', 'i', 'sh' and 's' are used as a quick check of how well the auditory system (i.e. the hearing plus hearing aids) is working. Each sound is different in pitch: 'm' very low (250 Hz), 'u' low (250–500 Hz), 'a' low-middle (750–1500 Hz), 'i' low and middle-high (250–500 and 2000–3000 Hz), 'sh' middle-high (2000+ Hz) and 's' high (4000+ Hz). When a child responds to all these sounds spoken at normal loudness, it tells us that he can detect the pitches important for listening to speech. Sometimes the test is used to check how well the child is able to discriminate these sounds (Ling, 1989). For example, the child who says 'u' in response to both 'u' and 'i' is not hearing enough of the middle-high frequencies to discriminate these vowels. The usefulness of this test depends on the sounds being presented at the same distance and loudness each time.

Chloe is now almost 5 and about to start in Year 1 at school. She has been in a resourced unit for the hearing impaired in a mainstream school since she was 3. She spends an increasing amount of time in the mainstream nursery. Chloe continues to be a strong-willed little girl, a good communicator with an inquisitive nature.

Sally thinks:

> We've been lucky with her because she has gone along and academically she's doing really well. She just wants to learn. She hasn't had to sign or anything like that which has been nice. I mean, obviously, it would have been different if she had had to sign. Then we would have learnt sign language but at the moment she doesn't need it. We feel now she can learn that when she is ready to. She is always going to be part of the deaf community so she can learn it when she feels she wants to.

Conclusion

Chloe is still profoundly hearing impaired, but the case study shows how she learnt to use every bit of the hearing she has. Learning to listen takes the dedication of parents and family, the support of an experienced audiology team and a responsive education service. It takes a long time and much effort, and everybody involved has to understand the implications of the hearing loss on the child and the family, and work together as a team.

Not every hearing impaired child will learn to listen and talk as readily as Chloe. There are many factors that affect a child's ability to make use of his residual hearing: his aided hearing levels, additional handicaps, 'intelligence', parental motivation and age when aided, for example. For some families, learning to listen and talk may not be a goal at all. Their goal may be for the child to become a confident communicator, but in sign language. Parents choose an auditory approach to communication when they judge that it offers their child greater opportunity in the hearing world.

Appendix: Auditory development – a checklist of auditory objectives

1. Shows an awareness of loud environmental sounds. (The child may show that he is aware of a sound in a variety of ways: by stilling, crying, stopping crying, eye blink, eye-widening, startling, changes in sucking, turning his head, looking up, pointing to his ear, saying 'Noise' and so on.)
2. Shows an awareness of voice:
   to a loud voice close by
   and a normal voice at 3–4 feet
3. Shows more responsiveness to 'motherese' than to adult–adult conversation. (The child may become more vocal or more active, make more eye contact and/or smile at the adult using 'motherese'.)
4. Shows an awareness of his own voice by becoming noisier.
5. Responds differently to angry and friendly voices. (The child may cry or frown when hearing angry voices.)
6. Responds differently to singing than to talking. (May be soothed by singing but not by talking.)
7. Enjoys making a noise with anything to hand.
8. Recognizes his mother's and father's voices. (May follow the conversation between his mother and father by looking at the one who is speaking.)
9. Recognizes some environmental sounds. (The child shows in some way that he knows what is making the noise; for example he goes to watch the washing machine when he hears it spinning.)
10. Recognizes some noise-making toys. (May search for the toy when he hears its sound.)
11. Dances or rocks in response to hearing music.
12. Associates an animal or toy sound with object. (For example, the adult says 'Where's the meow?', and the child looks at the cat.)
13. Shows recognition of a song/finger rhyme or a phrase by making a hand movement. (The child may wave a hand when the adult says 'Bye bye', or put out his hand in response to 'Let's do "Round and Round the Garden"'.)
14. Understands the words 'Mummy' and 'Daddy'; i.e. looks at his mother in response to 'Where's Mummy?'
15. Responds when his own name is called: from close by, from 6 feet away and from across the room.
16. Shows he understands the significance of some environmental sounds, for example looking expectantly at the door when someone is knocking or saying 'aaaaa' when Concorde is flying over the house.
17. Shows he is understanding frequently heard phrases when they are supported by context, for example 'Go and find your shoes' when getting ready to go out.
18. Recognizes his favourite finger plays and songs by joining in singing or with the actions.
19. Shows an understanding of single words in a carrier phrase, for example 'Find your ball' or 'Where's your nose?'

20. Listens to music and knows when it is on and off; for example, plays musical bumps.
21. Co-operates with play audiometry, usually between 24 and 36 months of age.

References

Aslin R, Pisoni D, Jusczyk P (1983) Auditory development and speech perception in infancy. In Haith M, Campos J (Eds) Handbook of Child Psychology, Vol. 2: Infancy and Developmental Psychobiology. New York: John Wiley & Sons.

Cole E (1992) Listening and Talking: A Guide to Promoting Spoken Language in Young Hearing-impaired Children. Washington, DC: AG Bell Association for the Deaf.

Crago MB, Erics-Brophy AA. (1993) Feeling Right: Approaches to a Family's Culture in Beginning with Babies: A Sharing of professional experience. Ling Phillips A, Coles EB (Eds) The Volta Review 95(5) November 1993..

Cross TG (1977) Mothers' speech adjustments: the contribution of selected child listener variables. In Snow CE, Ferguson CA (Eds) Talking to Children: Language Input and Acquisition. Cambridge: Cambridge University Press.

DeCasper A, Fifer W (1980) Of human bonding: newborns prefer their mothers' voices. Science 208: 1174–6.

Estabrooks W (1994) Auditory-verbal Therapy for Parents and Professionals. Washington, DC: AG Bell Association for the Deaf.

Fraiberg S (1979) Blind infants and their mothers: an examination of the sign system. In Bullowa M (Ed) Before Speech. Cambridge, Cambridge University Press.

Kingsley EP (1991) Kids like these. In Luterman DM, Ross M (Eds) When Your Child is Deaf, a Guide for Parents. Parkton, Maryland: York Press.

Lincoln & Louth NHS Trust (1996) Breaking Bad News. Guidelines for Best Practice. Lincoln: Lincoln & Louth NHS Trust.

Ling D (1989) Foundations of Spoken Language for Hearing-impaired Children. Washington, DC: AG Bell Association for the Deaf.

Oller DK, Eilers RE (1988) The role of audition in infant babbling. Child Development 59: 441–9.

Tucker B (1995) The Feel of Silence. Philadelphia: Temple University Press.

Watson L, Lewis S (1997) Working with parents: setting the parameters. Journal of British Association of Teachers of the Deaf 21(2): 32–40.

Useful addresses

Alexander Graham Bell Association of the Deaf
3417 Volta Place NW Washington DC 20007-2778, USA
Tel: +(202) 337 5220
Fax: +(202) 337 8270
e-mail: agbell2@aol.com

Auditory-Verbal International Inc.
2121 Eisenhower Avenue Suite 402
Alexandria VA 22314, USA
Tel: +703 739 1049
TDD: +703 739 0874
Fax: +703 739 0395
e-mail: avi@auditory-verbal.org

Glossary

Acoustic: relating to sound.

Acoustic reflex: middle ear muscle reflex in response to a loud sound.

Acute: short and relatively severe.

Aetiology: the origin, causation and development of disease.

Aided: pertaining to hearing as improved by a hearing aid

Ambient noise: background noise within a room or area

Anoxia: an absence or deficiency of oxygen reaching body tissue

Articulation: movement of tongue and lips and jaw to make sounds.

At risk: having greater than average chances of an impairment.

Attenuation: a reduction or weakening.

Audiogram: a chart showing an individual's hearing thresholds.

Audiometer: the instrument used to measure hearing.

Audiometry: the measurement of hearing using calibrated electronic instruments.

Audition: the sense of hearing.

Auditory perception: the ability to use hearing to perceive spoken language. It includes skills such as attention to sound, long and short term memory for sound, localisation of sound etc.

Auditory Brainstem Response audiometry (ABR): the measurement of hearing in which brain activity is recorded, usually in response to middle-to-high frequency sounds.

Auditory nerve (Acoustic nerve): the nerve of hearing which connects the cochlea to the brain.

Auditory-Verbal communication: an approach to developing the deaf child's listening skills as the means to process spoken language and to talk.

Auditory-Oral communication approaches: these include The Natural Aural approach and Structured Oral approaches. These approaches are based on the knowledge that the majority of deaf children have sufficient hearing, through the use of appropriate audiological aids, to develop understanding of spoken language. It is expected that they will follow a similar process of language acquisition to that of hearing children.

Augmentative Communication Methods: these often make use of a symbol system such as Bliss, Rebus or Makaton or use objects of reference, which may be selected from a chart or a board, either mechanically or electronically, to form sentences.

Behavioural hearing tests: hearing tests where the child is required to respond in some way to a sound.

Behavioural observation audiometry (BOA): the assessment of hearing by observing a child's unconditioned responses, such as eye blink, to sounds presented at measured levels in a sound treated room.

Behind the ear (BTE) hearing aid/ postaural hearing aid: a hearing aid that rests behind the ear and attaches by a tube leading into the ear canal.

Bilateral hearing loss: a hearing loss in both ears.

Bilingual communication: children are educated using British Sign Language (BSL) and learn English as an additional language.

Binaural: both ears.

Body worn hearing aid: a hearing aid worn on the chest or clipped to a pocket or harness, with a lead connecting it to the receiver worn at the ear.

Bone anchored hearing aid: this is a special bone conduction hearing aid which is attached to the head by a small screw implanted into the skull.

Bone conduction: the way sound is conducted to the cochlea through the bones of the head.

Bone conduction hearing aid: a hearing aid that uses a bone vibrator pressed against the skull to transmit sound directly to the inner ear.

Bone conduction testing: in this test the sound is presented through a vibrator, or bone conductor, placed behind the ear and held in place by a headband. The sound goes directly into the inner ear and bypasses any blockage or problem in the middle ear. The hearing of the inner ear can then be measured.

British Sign Language (BSL): BSL is recognized as a language distinct from English. It is the sign language indigenous to the deaf community of Britain. It has been defined as a visual, gestural language in terms of both its perception and production. As it is perceived visually within space, signs can be combined simultaneously to convey meaning. Body and head posture, facial expression and lip movements all play a distinctive role in contributing to meaning.

Canal atresia: absence of an ear canal. Instead of a canal there is bone or cartilage, resulting in a conductive hearing loss.

Canal hearing aid: a hearing aid that fits mostly in the ear canal.

Caregiver: any adult who takes care of a child.

Chromosome: units of inheritance of which there are normally 46 in humans.

Chronic: lasting a long time.

Chronological age: age from date of birth.

Cochlea: the inner ear.

Cochlear implant programme: service including assessment, fitting and follow-up for people who are considering or using a cochlear implant.

Cochlear implant system: the full set of components worn by a cochlear implant user, including implantable package, speech processor, microphone, transmitter coil and accessories.

Cochlear implant: a device surgically implanted into the inner ear which gives a sensation of sound through electrical stimulation of the auditory nerve.

Comfort zone: the area on an audiogram between the child's threshold and his loudness discomfort level.

Comprehension: attaching meaning to a given sound or word.

Conductive deafness: hearing loss caused by a problem in the outer or middle ear. It is often possible to correct conductive deafness with medicine or surgery.

Congenital: present at birth.

Consanguinity: close family relationship.

Cooing: vowel-like sounds made by a baby between 0 and 4 months.

CT (Computerized Tomography) scan: used for imaging of the inner ear as part of the assessment for cochlear implant surgery.

Cued speech: a one handed supplement to spoken language devised to clarify the phonemes of spoken language that are ambiguous or invisible in lip-reading.

Cytomegalovirus: a viral infection that can cause severe problems in the newborn including hearing loss.

Deaf: when written with an upper case 'D' is now a widely accepted way of denoting cultural deafness and describes people who elect to identify with the Deaf community, who choose most of their significant social contact within a Deaf group and who communicate through sign language.

deaf: when written with a lower case 'd' refers to anyone with a significant hearing loss.

Deaf Community: members of the Deaf Community perceive themselves to be a cultural and linguistic minority rather than a disabled group.

Decibel (dB): the unit for measuring the intensity of a sound. dB scales are logarithmic, that is to say that an apparently small difference of a few decibels can actually be a large difference in terms of sound energy. The decibel system allows workers in audiology and acoustics to describe, and deal with sound levels where the highest level which can be tolerated is around 10,000,000 times greater than the lowest level which normal ears can detect.

dBSPL(dB Sound Pressure Level): sound is effectively a rapid variation or vibration in pressure, and most of the time we are concerned with sound travelling in air. dB Sound Pressure Level is the way of describing sound levels in comparison with an extremely small level of air pressure variation which has been given the value of zero dBSPL. All sound measurements in dBSPL are referenced to this starting level. In physical terms this reference level is a pressure of $2\times10\text{-}5\text{N}/\text{m}2$.

dBA (dB A weighted): sound level meters can be set to measure sound in different ways for differing purposes. The 'A' weighting system allows the meter to react to sound in a similar way to the human ear, and sound levels in dBA are widely used in respect of the way sound affects people.

dBHL (dB Hearing level): dB Hearing Level is another special way of using the decibel when hearing is being measured. The dBHL system takes into account the differing sensitivity of the human ear to different pitches of sound. Puretone audiometry using headphones is always recorded in dBHL, and hearing tests in sound field rooms are usually measured in dBHL for convenient comparison.

Desired Sensation Level (DSL): this is a 'prescription' approach to determining what a hearing aid should do based on the child's hearing levels.

Developmental age: state of childhood development - not necessarily the same as the chronological age.

Digital hearing aids: the latest and most promising type of hearing aids where the programming and amplification are controlled by digital electronics.

Discrimination (auditory): perceiving differences in two unlike sounds.

Distraction testing: a technique for testing hearing in young children from about 6 months of age. Sounds are made behind the child while he plays quietly and if he hears the sound he turns to locate it. The sounds can be varied by frequency and intensity.

Ear impression taking: the first stage in the process of manufacturing an earmould. Soft impression material is syringed into the ear canal to obtain an accurate replica of the child's ear. When the impression has hardened it is gently removed and sent to a laboratory for manufacture.

Earmould: the plastic ear piece, specially made to fit the user's ear, which channels sound from the hearing aid into the ear canal.

Electro-acoustic analysis of hearing aids: this test forms part of the routine hearing aid review. The hearing aid's performance is accurately measured in a hearing aid test box or analyser. This allows comparison to be made with the manufacturer's specifications and to determine how the aid performs at the user's settings.

Electrocardiogram (ECG): a means of measuring the electrical activity of the heart.

Electrode array: wires surgically implanted in the inner ear which deliver electrical stimulation to the auditory nerve of a cochlear implant user.

ENT consultant: Ear, Nose and Throat specialist.

Environmental sounds: all sounds that occur in a given environment – not usually speech sounds unless specifically included.

Eustachian tube: a small tube that connects the middle ear to the back of the throat. It allows air into the middle ear and equalizes the pressure with the air outside.

Expressive language: symbolic communication using speech and/or signs.

Feedback: 1.(acoustic feedback) a whistling/squealing sound from the hearing aid which is due to the amplified sound leaking from the earmould and going back into the microphone. 2. The receipt of sensory information which allows a person to maintain or modify his performance.

Fingerspelling: Fingerspelling is the manual representation of the letters of the alphabet by 26 different hand positions. In the UK this is accomplished by means of a two handed alphabet but other variants exist.

Free-field test: a test of hearing where sounds are presented through loudspeakers in a sound treated room.

Frequency: the number of times, per second, a sound wave vibrates, measured in hertz (Hz).

Fricatives: speech sounds such as /f/ and /s/ that have turbulent breath flow.

Gain: the amount that a hearing aid amplifies sound. Gain is expressed in decibels.

Genetic counselling: a means of helping families where a hereditary cause for the hearing loss is suspected, to understand the probable pattern of inheritance.

Glue ear: fluid build up in the middle ear space behind the eardrum. This usually causes a mild and temporary hearing loss.

Grommet: a small tube inserted into the eardrum to keep the middle ear dry and free of fluid.

Habilitation: the process of supporting the family and hearing impaired child in adapting to hearing loss, becoming familiar with the hearing device and developing the child's communication skills.

Hair cells: the sensory receptor cells for hearing found within the cochlea.

Headset: ear level microphone and transmitter coil used with the body-worn speech processor of a cochlear implant system.

Health visitor (hearing) test: screening of babies for hearing loss, performed by health visitors, at around 8 months of age, using the distraction test.

Hearing age: the number of years a child has worn hearing aids or received stimulation from a cochlear implant.

Hearing aid: an electronic device to amplify sound worn in the ear or on the body.

Hearing Impaired: those with any degree of hearing loss from mild to profound.

Hertz: the unit for measuring the frequency of a sound.

Hyperacusis: a reduced tolerance to loud noise.

Impedance testing: this test measures the stiffness of the eardrum under different conditions of pressure. The change in stiffness is plotted on a chart called a tympanogram. In its main form, it is used not to test hearing but to check the whether the middle ear is working normally.

In-The-Ear (ITE) hearing aid: hearing aid in which the amplifier is built into the earmould so the whole hearing aid sits in the ear.

Individual Education Plan (IEP): a plan which sets out detailed targets and programmes for the hearing impaired pupil and success criteria against which progress will be judged.

Inner ear (cochlea): a small 'snail-like' structure containing a complex network of many thousands of sound sensitive cells.

Insert earphone: a small earphone which connects to an earmould that is inserted in the ear canal. This is an important tool in making ear-specific measurements on young children.

Intelligibility: the degree to which speech can be understood.

Intonation: variation in voice pitch during speech which gives its tuneful quality.

Intensity: the measured loudness of a sound, usually in decibels (dB).

Iris: coloured part of the eye.

Jargon: vocalisations (or hand movements) which sound like (or resemble) sentences but which have only occasional intelligible words (signs) interjected.

Jaundice: a condition in which the body becomes yellow as a result of deposits of bile pigment (bilirubin) in the body tissue.

kHz Kilohertz: 1000 hertz or cycles per second.

Loudness discomfort level (LDL): the amplified level of sound, usually speech, which the listener finds too loud.

LEA: Local Education Authority

Lexicon: vocabulary.

Lip-reading (Speech reading): this is the understanding of speech through the recognition of the facial patterns of different phonemes and groups of phonemes forming words. Good language levels will usually aid the ability to lip-read.

Literacy: the ability to read and write.

Localization: the determination of the apparent direction and/or distance of a sound source.

McCormick Toy Test: a speech discrimination test for use with children.

Mainstream schools: the schools catering for the majority of children.

Makaton Vocabulary: this comprises a specially selected vocabulary (taken from BSL) to provide a basis for communication often with children with severe learning difficulties. It is structured in stages of increasing complexity and follows the normal pattern of language development. The initial stages comprise basic vocabulary necessary to express some essential needs. Subsequent stages include more complex language.

Meatus: the ear canal.

Meningitis: inflammation of the membranes covering the brain and spinal chord. Meningitis is the main cause of permanent acquired hearing loss in children.

Middle ear: is the air filled cavity that contains three tiny bones (ossicles).

Mild hearing loss: an average hearing loss between 250 and 4000Hz of 20– 40 dBHL.

Mixed hearing loss: a loss which has a sensorineural and a conductive component.

Modelling: teaching behaviour through demonstration or use.

Moderate hearing loss: an average hearing loss between 250 and 4000Hz of 41–70 dBHL

Monaural: of or for only one ear.

Motherese: the way that many mothers and caregivers talk with small children.

MRI (Magnetic Resonance Imaging) scan: used for imaging of the inner ear as part of the assessment for cochlear implant surgery.

Myringotomy: surgical procedure to withdraw excess fluid from the middle ear.

National Literacy Strategy: a major literacy initiative by the DfEE to improve reading and writing standards of all school pupils.

Neonate: an infant during the first few weeks of life.

Non-verbal: not related to words.

Normal hearing: an average hearing level between 250 and 4000Hz of 0–19 dBHL.

Objective hearing test: hearing test where the child is not required to actively respond to a sound.

OFSTED Report: an inspection report that identifies the strengths and weakness of the school and the qualifications and National Curriculum levels that its pupils have achieved.

Ophthalmologist: medical practitioner specializing in disorders of the eye.

Ossicles: the small bones in the middle ear.

Otitis Media with Effusion(OME): commonly known as 'glue ear'. The resulting hearing loss is conductive and usually temporary.

Otoacoustic emissions (OAE) test: this is frequently used to screen very young children for hearing loss. The test is so sensitive that even a slight hearing loss can be detected.The test equipment records a small echo which the cochlea, in a normal ear, generates in response to a click played directly into the ear canal.

Otology: the branch of medicine that deals with disorders of the ear.

Otoscope: an instrument for examining the ear canal and eardrum.

Ototoxic: potentially damaging to the ear.

Paediatrician: doctor specialising in children.

Paget Gorman Signed Speech (previously Paget-Gorman Systematic Sign Language, PGSS): a simultaneous grammatical representation of spoken English, for use as an aid to the teaching of language. The signs have been artificially developed within a logical system but do not correspond to BSL national or regional signs.

Partially hearing/hard of hearing: usually a mild to moderate loss.

Perforation: hole

Performance testing: type of hearing test where the child performs a simple task whenever he hears a sound. This is most successful from two and a half years.

Perinatal: around the time of birth.

Peripatetic: travelling. Peripatetic teachers of the deaf travel to schools where hearing-impaired children are integrated and offer specialized advice and support to the mainstream classroom teachers. They also teach the hearing impaired children individually.

Pharynx: the area at the back of the mouth.

Pinna: the outer ear.

Postaural hearing aids: hearing aids worn behind the ear (BTE aids).

Postnatal: after birth.

Puretone audiometry: measurement of hearing using headphones, where frequency-specific and ear-specific information can be obtained and a pure tone audiogram (PTA) can be recorded.

Prelingual: before the development of language, or before 3 years of age.

Prelinguistic (presymbolic) communication: the way an infant or child conveys his feeling, wants and needs before s/he can talk. It includes behaviours such as crying, body movements, body posture, eye contact, gazing, touching, pointing, and pulling on an object or a person.

Prenatal: before birth

Probe tube: small tube with microphone for measuring sound pressure levels in the ear.

Profound hearing loss: an average hearing loss between 250 and 4000Hz of more than 95dBHL.

Programming (also tuning, mapping, fitting): process by which the required levels of electrical stimulation are determined, and the speech processor adjusted, for the individual cochlear implant user.

Progressive hearing loss: becoming worse over time.

Pure tone average (PTA): the average of hearing thresholds at the frequencies 500Hz, 1000Hz, 2000Hz and 4000Hz for each ear.

Radio hearing aid (FM system): a system where the mother or teacher wears a microphone and a FM (frequency modulated) transmitter. The child wears a FM receiver which picks up sound directly from the transmitter microphone. This system goes some way to reducing the problem of background noise.

Real-ear measurements: a means of measuring the amplification produced by a hearing aid in a child's ear by means of a probe microphone.

Receptive language: the symbols (words, signs) understood by a person.

Recruitment: an abnormally rapid growth in the sensation of loudness, such that sounds quickly become uncomfortably loud. This problem often accompanies cochlear damage.

Reduplicated babble: using consonant-vowel syllable repetitions e.g. ma-ma-ma-ma.

Resource base (sometimes called specialist units, partially hearing units, units for the hearing impaired): special classroom(s) within mainstreamed schools which have extra resources, training and equipment, and the services of one or more qualified teachers of the deaf and other trained personnel.

Residual hearing: the auditory abilities of a person with a hearing impairment.

Respite care: short-term care for disabled children.

Retina: tissue at the back of the eye (necessary for vision).

Retrocochlear hearing loss: a hearing impairment due to problems in the pathways that transmit signals from the cochlea to the brain, or to damage within the brain itself.

Room acoustics: the way sound is affected by the characteristics of a room such as size and wall surface.

Screening for hearing impairment in children: giving a simple but sensitive test which children with normal hearing will pass and hearing impaired children will fail.

Sensorineural deafness: the impairment of hearing due to problems in the cochlear and/or the auditory nerve.

Severe hearing loss: an average hearing loss between 250 and 4000Hz of 71-95 dBHL.

Sign communication approach: some children use sign for part or all of their time in education; some will choose to use sign as their principal method of communication throughout their lives.

Sign Supported English: a manual support system incorporating signs from BSL together with finger spelling. It is used in English word order to supplement spoken words but does not attempt to present every element of the spoken utterance. Its aim is to clarify the spoken message and lessen ambiguity.

Signed English (British): signs taken from BSL together with generated signs and markers, are used, with fingerspelling to give an exact manual representation of spoken English. It is used primarily as a tool for the teaching of reading and writing.

Sound field: the area within a sound-treated room.

Speech discrimination testing: measures the ability to hear the differences between sounds in speech.

Special Educational Needs (SEN): the 1993 Education Act defines a child as having special educational needs (SEN) if 'he or she has a learning difficulty which calls for special educational provision to be made for him or her.'

Specialist schools for the deaf: currently there are approximately 40 specialist schools for the deaf in the United Kingdom, many of which specialize in supporting deaf children with particular learning needs, who need a particular approach to language acquisition and communication and who are of a particular age or ability range.

Speech processor: component of the cochlear implant system which encodes sounds as patterns of electrical stimulation which will be delivered by the implanted electrode array to the auditory nerve.

Sporadic: condition occurring in isolated cases.

Statement of Special Educational Need: this is a formal document which identifies the child's special needs and legally binds the local education authority to meet these needs.

Switch-on: term used to describe the initial fitting of a cochlear implant speech processor. This term can be rather misleading as initial programming with young children is a gradual process.

Symbolic language: the use of an orderly arrangement of symbols – spoken words, sign language, or written words – to convey meaning.

Syndrome: a number of symptoms that collectively indicate a specific abnormality.

Syntax: the system of rules governing the creation of sentences.

Tactile: to do with the sense of touch.

Targeted Neonatal Screening: test at birth of babies who are most at risk for deafness.

Threshold of hearing: the intensity at which a person can just barely detect a given sound. This may be measured with the aids in place-aided, or without the aids – unaided.

Total Communication: there is variation in its interpretation and use. It is seen as a flexible approach to communication in which children may vary in how they receive and express language. Therefore, in those establishments which espouse a TC approach, a variety of different models may be used, e.g. aural/oral communication, BSL, SSE, fingerspelling.

Tympanic membrane: the eardrum.

Unilateral hearing loss: a hearing loss in one ear.

Unisensory: involving only one sense.

Universal neonatal screening (for hearing loss): test at birth of all babies in the district.

Verbal: related to words, spoken or written.

Vestibular system: the balance system which is connected to the cochlea.

Vibrotactile: sounds which are felt rather than heard.

Vocalizations: babbling sounds produced by infants.

Visual reinforcement audiometry (VRA): in this test of hearing sounds are presented from one side of the child. When the child turns to look he is given a visual reward such as a teddy bear with eyes flashing. This test works well from 6 months of age.

Index

Printed and bound by CPI Group (UK) Ltd, Croydon, CR0 4YY

27/10/2024

14580141-0005